The Anti-Hustle Health Plan: How to Get Fit, Stay Sane, and Actually Enjoy Your Life

A Lazy Genius Guide to Wellness for Overachievers,

Burnouts, and People Who Hate the Gym

Dr. Ben Chuba
&
Nicci Brochard

The Anti-Hustle Health Plan: How to Get Fit, Stay Sane, and Actually Enjoy Your Life

A Lazy Genius Guide to Wellness for Overachievers,

Burnouts, and People Who Hate the Gym

For permissions, licensing, or inquiries, please contact

info@crossborderpublishers.com: www.crossborderpublishers.com

Book Formatting by: Monisha

Book cover design by: *Billy Design*

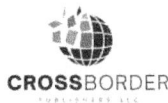

CROSSBORDER

New York, London, Quebec

Contents

Introduction

In the rush to achieve, we often forget the most important thing: enjoying life along the way. We've been conditioned to believe that fitness and wellness must be strenuous, relentless, and perfectly executed, or else we're failing. But what if getting fit, staying sane, and actually enjoying life didn't require endless hours at the gym or an unsustainable obsession with perfection?

Welcome to *The Anti-Hustle Health Plan*. This isn't your typical wellness book with rigid diets, extreme workouts, or the pressure to always do more. Instead, it's a laid-back, intelligent guide designed for overachievers, burnouts, and those who can't imagine another soul-crushing treadmill session. You can still get healthier, stronger, and more energized—all without sacrificing your sanity or time.

This plan isn't about squeezing fitness into an already overloaded life. It's about redefining wellness to fit *you*. Through simple strategies, grounded science, and a refreshing mindset, we'll show you how to move well, eat intuitively, rest deeply, and, most importantly, reclaim the joy that's so often lost in the hustle.

It's time to stop battling against your body and start working with it. With a little creativity and some well-chosen habits, you'll feel better, move better, and live better—without ever needing to turn your life upside down. So take a deep breath, let go of the guilt, and let's start making wellness work for you, not against you. You've got this.

Ben and I (Nicci) thank you immensely for choosing our book. We promise you a great time ahead.

Chapter 1

The Hustle Trap and Burnout

Hustle Culture Hangover

"*If you want to get better, you have to work harder—no excuses, no days off.*" This mantra of the modern grind is glorified on social media and echoed in offices and gyms alike. But what happens after the adrenaline of constant hustle wears off? Many high-achievers find themselves in a *hustle culture hangover* – mentally and physically exhausted, yet guilt-ridden if they dare slow down. They push through fatigue, convinced that relentless effort is the only path to success. Ironically, research shows the opposite: excessive work or exercise without rest leads to diminishing returns. A Harvard Business Review analysis famously concluded that chronic overwork becomes "a story of diminishing returns: keep overworking, and you'll progressively work more stupidly on tasks that are increasingly meaningless". In other words, beyond a certain point, each additional hour of grinding yields less and less – or even negative – productivity. The same holds true for fitness; powering through workouts on fumes can stall progress. Trainers note that the idea of pushing through exhaustion as a badge of honor is misguided – sometimes *skipping* a workout to rest is actually the smarter choice. When you are sleep-deprived and drained, your muscles don't recover, your form suffers, and you risk injury and burnout. Prioritizing rest is not laziness; it's physiology and common sense. One sports nutritionist

3

explains that if you consistently exercise on little sleep, you'll end up perpetually tired, and performance and health will decline. In short, the "no excuses" grind mindset can backfire badly. Instead of viewing rest as weakness, we must recognize it as a critical component of sustainable improvement – the secret sauce that the hustle hype forgot.

The hustle hangover is most obvious in the aftermath of an all-out sprint: the entrepreneur who hasn't taken a day off in months, or the fitness buff who refuses to schedule rest days. Initially, they might see gains – a burst of productivity, a spike in strength – but soon fatigue accumulates. The body and mind start to rebel. Studies on overtraining in athletes find that relentless training without rest elevates cortisol (the stress hormone), weakens the immune system, and increases injury risk. Similarly, professionals logging 70–80 hour workweeks discover that beyond ~50 hours, their output actually drops. One professor who tracked his own work hours found that when he pushed past 50 hours a week, his productivity declined and mistakes multiplied. In extreme cases, managers can't even tell the difference between employees working 80-hour weeks and those just *pretending* to do so – a striking illustration that endless hustle often just produces *the appearance* of productivity, not real results. The human brain and body have limits. Caffeine and willpower might prop you up for a while, but at a certain point, exhaustion exacts its toll: concentration wavers, creativity plummets, and you start "working more stupidly" on those long to-do lists. What's more, being **always on** carries an opportunity cost – time not spent sleeping, relaxing, or connecting with others is time your body and mind can't recover. That recovery isn't optional; it's when muscles rebuild, memories consolidate, and stress hormones rebalance. Skipping it, as the hustle culture encourages, leads straight to the burnout trap.

When Success Sabotages Health

There is a cruel paradox in modern culture: the people who *"have it all"* on paper – high-powered careers, successful businesses, disciplined routines – are often privately falling apart. When professional or academic success is achieved by sacrificing sleep, mental health, and downtime, the victory can be pyrrhic. Chronic stress and burnout begin to sabotage health in serious ways, underscoring the need for a new approach to "success." Consider the evidence: long-term job burnout and stress are strongly linked to some of the very health problems we most fear. For example, extensive studies in Europe found that working consistently beyond 55 hours per week raises the risk of stroke by 33% and the risk of heart attack by 13%, compared to a more reasonable 35–40 hour workweek. The Finnish Institute of Occupational Health reported that the stress of overwork can trigger a cascade of issues – depression, impaired sleep, memory problems, even heart disease. It's not just anecdotal; it's biochemical. Chronic stress elevates blood pressure and cortisol levels, disrupts blood sugar regulation, and promotes inflammation – over time, this contributes to hypertension, cardiovascular disease, and yes, even diabetes. A recent study presented at an American Heart Association conference found that women with the highest levels of chronic stress had nearly double the risk of developing type 2 diabetes. In other words, the hormonal and metabolic fallout from constant pressure can literally alter the course of your health.

And perhaps unsurprisingly, burnout often comes hand-in-hand with insomnia or troubled sleep. Research shows that burnout and insomnia feed each other in a vicious cycle – stress keeps you awake, and sleepless nights make you more vulnerable to stress. Many overwhelmed high-achievers find themselves tired but *wired*, unable to shut off racing thoughts at night. This loss of restorative sleep then exacerbates fatigue, brain fog, and emotional volatility during the day.

It's sobering to realize that the badge of honor we call "hard work" can mask a slow-motion health crisis. The executive pulling all-nighters may see short-term wins, but over time their immune system might weaken, their waistline might expand (stress eating and cortisol can encourage fat storage), and their doctor may start warning about high blood sugar or cholesterol. Medical literature now speaks of "overachievement at the cost of health" as a genuine phenomenon: Type-A individuals driving themselves into chronic illness. For instance, one long-term study found that work stress is an independent risk factor for type 2 diabetes, especially in women. Another showed that persistent job strain and long hours correlate with poorer sleep quality and higher incidence of insomnia symptoms. We also know severe burnout can manifest psychologically with anxiety, depression, or a sense of detachment – the classic burnout profile of emotional exhaustion and cynicism. In sum, the human body will only endure so much relentless pressure before it starts to break down. Heart disease, diabetes, and insomnia are just a few of the red flags waving at us to change course. If success is coming at the expense of your health, is it really success at all? This question sets the stage for why an *anti-hustle* health plan is desperately needed. The very drive that helped you achieve goals can turn into self-sabotage if it is not balanced with self-care. Recognizing this paradox is the first step: winning in one arena (work, career, achievement) does not compensate for *losing* your wellness. The good news is that this trade-off isn't inevitable – it's possible to excel without burning out, but it requires rejecting the false idol of constant hustle and rethinking our definition of "hard work."

Why We Hate the Gym

Given all the above, one would think exercise should be a welcome stress-reliever – a chance to boost health and undo some of hustle culture's damage. So why do so many busy, burned-out people absolutely *dread* the gym? The reality is that traditional exercise routines often fail the very people who need them most. Let's unpack this candidly: many high-performing individuals simply hate the gym. They hate the slog, the boredom, the awkwardness, or the feeling that it's yet another obligation on an already packed schedule. One big factor is the *intimidating gym culture* that pervades many fitness spaces. Walking into a gym can feel like walking onto an unwelcome stage, especially if you're not already fit or confident. Surveys have found that about half of Americans feel too intimidated to even visit a gym and work out around others. They fear being judged – worrying that everyone is staring at their body or their performance. In one survey, nearly 2 in 5 people (39%) said they avoid exercise because they feel self-conscious about how they look. Even among those who do go to the gym, almost half admit they still feel uncomfortable exercising next to someone extremely fit. It's no wonder terms like "gymtimidation" have entered the lexicon. The very environment meant to encourage health can, paradoxically, make people feel inadequate or unwelcome. If you're an overachiever used to excelling at work, being a novice struggling on the treadmill in front of strangers can be an ego gut-punch. Many quietly decide it's not worth the anxiety.

Aside from social intimidation, there's the plain fact that conventional workouts often come across as *boring or punishing*. Dragging yourself through the same uninspired routine on the elliptical or lifting weights with no enjoyment can feel like a chore – yet another item on the to-do list. Psychology and exercise science tell us that this is a recipe for failure: enjoyment is actually one of the strongest predictors of sticking with exercise long-term. If you find workouts dull or dreadful, you're unlikely to keep doing them. Indeed, a study on exercise adherence noted that lack of interest or enjoyment is a commonly reported barrier, cited by roughly 1 in 5 people. Busy people who are already mentally exhausted from work have limited willpower reserves at the end of the day – convincing themselves to do something they hate (like an hour of tedious exercise) is a losing battle. Moreover, burnout comes with fatigue; feeling too tired is another top reason people skip workouts. In one large survey, more than 50% reported feelings of tiredness as a major barrier to being physically active. This is a cruel catch-22: you're exhausted from work, so you skip exercise; skipping exercise can make your energy and mood worse in the long run, but in the short run it's hard to overcome that inertia. Physiologically, chronic stress can sap motivation and make intense exercise feel especially hard – when you're already running on empty, a tough workout can send your brain a signal that it's *too much*.

Research confirms that sleep deprivation and high stress will diminish your exercise motivation and even your coordination, making injuries more likely if you do force yourself through a hard session. Little wonder that so many sincere New Year's resolutioners flame out by February. In fact, about 80% of people who join a gym in January quit within five weeks. Traditional fitness advice ("just do it," "no pain no gain") often fails these people by not addressing the root of the issue: the workouts are not enjoyable, not fitting into their busy lives, or not considerate of their mental state.

To truly help overachievers and burned-out folks embrace exercise, we have to acknowledge these psychological barriers. The gym might not be the *ideal* solution for everyone. Some might do better swapping competitive or high-pressure fitness environments for something gentler – like a solo walk in nature, a low-key yoga class, or even home workouts where they don't feel judged. Others need variety and fun: dance classes, sports, or "exercise snacks" (short bouts of activity) to keep boredom at bay. Behavioral scientists note that aligning exercise with personal preferences and pleasure – rather than treating it as self-punishment – is key to consistency. And crucially, any regimen must account for limited time and energy. For a busy professional, a realistic plan might be finding a 20-minute routine that energizes rather than exhausts, instead of insisting on a 90-minute gym session that just isn't going to happen on a hectic day. The bottom line is that if you've ever said "I hate the gym," you're far from alone. There are valid reasons so many feel that way, from gymtimidation to mind-numbing workout plans. Recognizing these hurdles is the first step in crafting a new approach to fitness – one that doesn't drive people away, but draws them in even when life is overwhelming.

The Call for an Anti-Hustle Revolution

It's clear by now that the prevailing "hustle hard" approach to wellness isn't working for a huge segment of people. The evidence and lived experiences point to one conclusion: we need an anti-hustle revolution in health and fitness. This revolution champions a gentler, smarter, and more sustainable philosophy – one that helps people get fit and stay sane *without* burning out or hating their lives. What might this look like? For starters, it means rejecting the extremes. Science is on our side here. Cutting-edge research in exercise science suggests that you *don't* have to push yourself to the brink to see results. In fact, a study from the University of Alberta found that moderate-intensity exercise produces almost the same physical benefits as maximal intensity workouts, but with far fewer risks. The researchers concluded it's essentially about *working smarter, not harder*: exercising at a reasonable effort (around 6 out of 10 on an exertion scale) gives you the gains of exercise *while* keeping you fresh enough to stay consistent over time. The participants who went all-out hit a wall – they experienced extreme fatigue, high stress hormone levels, and even nausea, which undermined their motivation to continue. Those who exercised more moderately were able to sustain their routine and felt better overall. This reinforces a pivotal idea for the anti-hustle approach: maximum effort is not the goal; consistency and sustainability are. You're better off doing a 30-minute moderate workout three times a week than a killer 2-hour session once in a blue moon that leaves you so sore and miserable you never want to return. Fitness, like success, is a marathon, not a sprint.

The anti-hustle philosophy also emphasizes recovery and mental well-being as non-negotiable parts of the plan. In the context of exercise, that means valuing rest days *as much as* workout days. Far from losing progress, smart rest actually *accelerates* improvement by allowing the body to repair and come back stronger. Sports medicine studies show that endurance adaptations (like stronger muscles and better cardiovascular fitness) occur primarily during rest – not during the workout itself. Even elite athletes incorporate rest, and research suggests you won't lose fitness after a single day or even a week off; on the contrary, strategic downtime can enhance performance. In an anti-hustle wellness plan, sleep, rest, and leisure aren't "wasted time" – they are active ingredients in your health, equally as important as the work you put in. This is corroborated by neuroscience and psychology: adequate sleep dramatically improves learning, mood, and motivation to exercise, whereas chronic sleep deprivation erodes willpower and increases anxiety. In one telling example, when basketball players in a Stanford study extended their sleep to ~10 hours a night, their sprint times and shooting accuracy significantly improved. Rest is the secret weapon that hustle culture forgot.

Another pillar of the anti-hustle revolution is making wellness enjoyable and personalized. We've seen that forcing yourself into a cookie-cutter diet or exercise plan that you despise is a dead end. The "lazy genius" approach, as we might call it, means finding clever, individualized ways to be healthy that don't feel like torture. It's about doing the *minimum effective dose* needed for benefit and choosing activities that deliver a high return on enjoyment and results for the time invested. Psychology research underscores that when physical activity is linked to personal enjoyment – say you love biking outdoors or you have fun playing pick-up soccer – your adherence skyrockets. On the flip side, if you're exercising solely out of guilt or to "burn calories" without any intrinsic satisfaction, you're unlikely to keep it up. Thus, the anti-hustle method encourages people to experiment and find what forms of movement they actually like (or at least don't hate). It might be unconventional: maybe walking meetings during work, or doing ten-minute yoga stretches in your pajamas, or gardening, or dancing in your living room. If it gets you moving and relieves stress, it counts. This approach also recognizes the power of self-compassion over self-criticism. Instead of berating yourself for not pushing hard enough, the new ethos says: celebrate any positive step, no matter how small. Skipped the gym because you were exhausted? In the old mindset, you'd feel like a failure. In the new mindset, you acknowledge you listened to your body and maybe took a relaxing walk instead – which likely did more for your wellbeing that day. Ironically, research shows that being kind to oneself about slip-ups can reduce stress and help people resume healthy behaviors faster than a cycle of guilt and shame.

In summary, the call for an anti-hustle revolution is a call to rebalance. It asks us to blend achievement with enjoyment, effort with recovery, ambition with compassion. This doesn't mean abandoning goals or becoming lazy – it means being a "lazy genius," using smarter strategy in place of sheer force of will. You can still get fit, write that book, get the promotion – but you can do it in a way that doesn't destroy your sanity or health. This chapter has highlighted why the current hustle trap leads to burnout and why so many struggle with traditional fitness. From here, we pivot to a new vision: a wellness philosophy grounded in science and common sense, where health and success complement rather than compete with each other. It's about time we redefine the grind and prove that taking care of yourself is not antithetical to high achievement – in fact, it might be the secret ingredient that makes success *sustainable*. The rest of this book will serve as a guide to this anti-hustle health plan, showing you how to get fit, stay sane, and actually enjoy your life while you do it. After all, life is too short (and our bodies too precious) for anything less.

Chapter 2

Redefining Wellness for Real Life

Ditching All-or-Nothing Thinking

One of the first mindsets to shed on the journey to realistic wellness is the all-or-nothing mentality. Too often, we fall into a trap of thinking that if we can't do something 100% perfectly, we shouldn't bother at all. This cognitive distortion plays out in familiar ways – for example, someone might say *"I've already blown my healthy eating today by having dessert, so I might as well eat all the cookies."* This "might as well" spiral wrecks our momentum and leaves us feeling defeated. Psychology experts note that such *all-or-none* thoughts are invalid and unhelpful, yet they can become automatic if we don't catch them. Instead of viewing one slip as a total failure, it's crucial to recognize these extremes as distortions and deliberately replace them with more flexible thinking.

Wellness is not a pass/fail exam. Embracing a moderate, sustainable approach can yield better results than drastic swings between overzealous effort and burnout. Research in behavioral health shows that rigid, perfectionistic thinking sets unrealistic expectations and is linked to anxiety, depression, and learned helplessness. In contrast, flexibility is a strength: being able to bend your plan when life happens means you won't break your healthy habits entirely. For instance, missing a workout or indulging at a party does not erase your progress; a flexible mindset lets you continue the next day without self-reproach. By seeing health as a *lifelong journey* rather than a binary success/failure, you build resilience. Each day becomes an opportunity to make small positive choices, not a verdict on your worth or willpower.

Importantly, consistency trumps intensity over the long run. A growing body of evidence suggests that small habits sustained daily can outshine intermittent extreme efforts. In one study, a group of sedentary adults was divided into two exercise regimens: one did brief high-intensity interval training (HIIT) three times a week, while the other did moderate-intensity exercise (like brisk cycling) five times a week. After several weeks, the moderate, frequent exercisers saw significant health improvements – lower body fat and better blood pressure – that *did not* show up in the infrequent HIIT group. In short, "slow, steady, and sustainable" outperformed the occasional all-out approach. The lead researcher noted that while any exercise is beneficial, doing something active almost every day was more effective for improving key health markers like blood pressure and blood sugar control. This finding reinforces a commonsense principle: you gain more by walking 30 minutes each day than by doing an exhausting two-hour workout once in a blue moon. Consistency builds habits, and habits compound over time.

We can apply this lesson broadly. Rather than overhauling your entire diet overnight or declaring you'll run a marathon next month, start with tiny, manageable changes. For example, commit to adding one serving of vegetables to your daily meals or taking the stairs instead of the elevator at work. These actions may seem minor, but done regularly, they add up to meaningful improvement. Crucially, they are *sustainable* — you're far more likely to stick with a 10-minute daily walk than a brutal bootcamp that leaves you sore for a week. Research on habit formation supports this incremental strategy: small successes build self-efficacy, making it easier to adopt further healthy behaviors, whereas extreme efforts often lead to injury or discouragement, causing people to give up entirely. Indeed, it's estimated that the majority of extreme New Year's fitness resolutions fizzle out within weeks, in large part because the changes are too drastic to maintain. By ditching the all-or-nothing mindset, you free yourself from that boom-and-bust cycle. Every healthy choice counts, and a misstep isn't catastrophic — it's just a detour on a very long road.

To illustrate, consider a case study of a busy professional named *Alex*. At one time, Alex approached wellness with an all-or-nothing attitude: either he would adhere to a strict, punishing diet and a 6-day-per-week intense gym schedule, or, if one thing went wrong, he'd abandon healthy habits completely. Unsurprisingly, this led to yo-yo results. He would be "all-in" for a few weeks, then inevitably life events or exhaustion would derail his plan — leading to guilt, binge eating, and sedentariness. Alex finally broke this cycle by reframing his efforts as continuous progress rather than perfect compliance. He set modest goals: eating a protein-rich breakfast each morning and taking a 20-minute walk at lunchtime. These were not dramatic changes, but he did them consistently, even on busy days. The small wins gave him energy and confidence to add more habits gradually. Over months, Alex lost weight and felt more energetic – not through any extreme program, but by showing up consistently for himself. His story underscores that wellness is built day by day. The "all or nothing" thinking had only sabotaged him, whereas embracing *"always something"* thinking kept him moving forward.

By challenging the notion that wellness has to be extreme, we redefine success. It's no longer "I failed because I missed two gym days this week"; instead it's "I succeeded because I exercised three days this week, and I'll try for four next week." This shift from a *binary* mindset to a *continuum* mindset is liberating. You begin to see health not as a destination (with an imagined perfect body or ideal benchmark) but as a continuous journey that will have ebbs and flows. In practice, this means focusing on doing the *right thing more often than not*, rather than doing the perfect thing all the time. Over the years, this approach delivers far greater dividends for your fitness, mental sanity, and self-esteem. Ultimately, by ditching all-or-nothing thinking, you give yourself permission to be human – to have good days and bad – while still moving in the direction of wellness. That patience and persistence will carry you much farther than any short-lived extreme ever could.

Wellness as Self-Care, Not Self-Punishment

Another crucial reframing is to view all your health practices – exercise, diet, sleep routines, etc. – as forms of self-care rather than as self-punishment. In a culture that often equates "working out" with *"working off"* indulgences, many people unconsciously adopt a negative motivation for fitness. We tell ourselves we must atone for eating that slice of cake by doing extra cardio, or that we don't deserve rest because we haven't been productive enough. This mindset turns wellness into a penance for not being "good enough," and it's profoundly demotivating and unsustainable. In fact, psychological research indicates that harsh self-criticism – while sometimes mistaken for a motivator – usually backfires. Beating yourself up mentally activates the brain's threat-defense system, triggering stress and a fight-or-flight response. When we feel under attack by our own inner voice, we are actually more likely to shut down, lose motivation, or seek comfort in unhealthy outlets (like overeating or alcohol). In other words, *viewing wellness as punishment creates a vicious cycle* of stress and failure, rather than the inspiration we hope for.

The good news is that the opposite approach — self-compassion — is not only kinder but far more effective at improving motivation and well-being. Self-care in wellness means treating yourself like you would a dear friend: with encouragement, patience, and understanding. If a friend said they felt bad for missing a workout, you wouldn't say "Yes, you're lazy and you'd better punish yourself tomorrow." More likely, you'd say "Don't be so hard on yourself, you'll get back on track – you're doing great overall!" Remarkably, offering ourselves this same kindness yields powerful benefits. Studies show that self-compassion breaks the cycle of stress that comes with perceived failures, making people more resilient after setbacks. Instead of drowning in guilt or shame, those who practice self-compassion can objectively acknowledge a lapse ("I didn't exercise this week") without self-condemnation, and then recommit to their goals calmly. This gentle mindset isn't about making excuses or "letting yourself off the hook" – it's about *motivating through care rather than fear.*

A growing body of research supports the idea that treating wellness as self-care leads to better outcomes. For example, sports psychologists have found that positive self-talk improves athletes' performance and confidence, while reducing anxiety. In the realm of personal health, a review of 79 studies (with over 16,000 participants) found that people who maintain a caring, positive attitude toward themselves in the face of failures tend to be happier and more successful in their goals. They experience greater well-being partly because they avoid the toxic guilt that paralyzes progress. In fact, an individual's level of self-compassion has been shown to predict mental health outcomes more strongly than many external factors – it can protect against anxiety and depression even more than things like a history of trauma or lack of social support. Clearly, being kind to yourself is not complacency; it's a smart strategy for long-term wellness. When you slip up, responding with understanding ("It's okay, I'm human, I'll try again tomorrow") keeps you in a growth mindset, ready to continue, instead of in a shame spiral that might make you quit.

There is also evidence that self-care-oriented motivation boosts perseverance. Pioneering researcher Dr. Kristin Neff and colleagues have documented that people who practice self-compassion tend to have *higher personal standards and more intrinsic motivation* – they strive for improvement out of genuine desire, not a feeling of worthlessness. They are also less afraid of failure and more likely to try again after a setback, because a failure doesn't devastate their self-image. By contrast, those who rely on self-criticism often become *more* afraid of failing (since every failure is tied to harsh judgment of their worth), which can lead to procrastination or giving up. In essence, self-compassionate people are in it for the long haul – they see taking care of their body and mind as an act of love, so they naturally want to continue, learn, and grow. Meanwhile, people who torture themselves with negative self-talk can burn out quickly or avoid challenges altogether, confirming their worst fears.

Consider the difference in two mindsets: "I must go to the gym because I ate junk – I hate how weak I am; if I don't push myself, I'm a failure" versus "I want to go to the gym to feel strong and energized – it's been a stressful day, so exercise will help me feel better." The first attitude is punitive, driven by self-loathing; the second is compassionate, driven by self-care. Over time, the person with the second attitude is far more likely to stick with exercise and reap its benefits. In fact, case studies in health coaching show that when individuals shift from a punishment paradigm to a self-care paradigm, their whole relationship with wellness changes. For example, a woman named *Jen* used to force herself on long runs out of guilt for her eating habits. She often described her workouts as "paying for my sins" and unsurprisingly, she dreaded exercising. After working with a coach, Jen learned to frame her runs as "me-time" – a chance to clear her head and boost her mood. She also gave herself permission to choose gentler activities (like yoga or walking) on days she felt exhausted, rather than seeing it as failure. The result? Jen actually *exercised more consistently* and found joy in it. By treating movement as a gift to herself rather than a punishment, she broke out of the cycle of dread and avoidance.

The takeaway is that nourishing your body and mind out of kindness is far more sustainable than whipping yourself into shape through scolding and shame. This doesn't mean you'll never skip a workout or eat something regrettable – it means when you do, you won't indulge a barrage of self-criticism. You can hold yourself accountable *without* cruelty. Indeed, top psychologists emphasize that taking responsibility for your actions works best when divorced from toxic guilt. You acknowledge a mistake, learn from it, and move on – just as you would forgive a friend and encourage them onward. By reorienting your motivation to self-care, every healthy choice becomes an act of self-respect and compassion. You start exercising because it relieves your stress, eating better because it fuels a clearer mind, sleeping well because you deserve rest – not because you're "not enough" and need to fix yourself. Ironically, when you stop using wellness habits as punishment, you remove the dread and resistance around them, making it *more enjoyable* to keep doing those habits. Over time, this positive cycle reinforces itself: self-care leads to feeling better, which motivates more self-care. Science and experience both confirm that being kind to yourself is a powerful catalyst for real change – far more than being your own drill sergeant ever could be.

The Lazy Genius Philosophy: Focus on What Matters

In the modern world of wellness, there's no shortage of advice. We are bombarded with tips on optimizing every aspect of our health – from 12-step morning routines to exotic superfoods and cutting-edge biohacks. It's easy to feel that *being healthy* requires doing all the things, all the time. This is where the "Lazy Genius" philosophy offers a breath of fresh air. Coined by author Kendra Adachi, the idea is to "be a genius about what matters and lazy about what doesn't." In other words, identify the small subset of habits that yield the majority of benefits, and focus your energy on those – unapologetically neglecting the rest. Applied to wellness, this means embracing the Pareto Principle (the 80/20 rule): roughly 20% of actions may account for 80% of your results. By concentrating on that vital 20%, you maximize your health gains without exhausting yourself on minutiae. This approach is perfect for overachievers and burnt-out folks who feel they "should" be doing everything; it gives permission to do less, but smarter.

What might those high-impact habits be? While it can vary slightly from person to person, a vast amount of research in public health points to a core set of fundamentals that disproportionately influence our well-being. In fact, a landmark analysis by Harvard scientists found that just five basic lifestyle habits could extend lifespan by over a decade on average. These were the common-sense pillars of health: eating a nutritious diet, exercising regularly, maintaining a healthy body weight, not smoking, and moderating alcohol intake. Participants who consistently did those five things had an 82% lower risk of dying from heart disease and significantly lower risk of cancer compared to those who did none. The dramatic findings suggest that *most* of the variance in long-term health comes down to a few simple behaviors. In other words, if you get the basics right, you reap enormous benefits. By contrast, obsessing over minor tweaks (like a trendy supplement or the perfect brand of running shoes) yields only marginal gains. This isn't to say the smaller things never matter, but rather that your physical and mental resources are limited – so you should spend them where they count most.

To be a "lazy genius" in wellness, start by figuring out which habits move *your* needle the most. Often, improving sleep is a top candidate. For many, getting a full 7–8 hours of quality sleep each night will do more for their mood, metabolism, and cognitive function than any fancy diet or workout plan. If you are chronically sleep-deprived, that one factor alone can undermine every other wellness effort; conversely, fixing your sleep can make healthy eating and exercise feel exponentially easier because you aren't running on empty. Nutrition is another high-impact area: simply shifting to eating mostly whole, minimally-processed foods (think vegetables, fruits, lean proteins, whole grains, healthy fats) and cutting back on excess sugar and ultra-processed snacks can transform key health markers like blood pressure, blood sugar, and energy levels. You don't need a perfect diet – just focus on real, nourishing foods most of the time (some experts literally recommend an "80/20" approach to eating, where 80% of your meals are healthy and 20% are treats or less ideal foods, to maintain balance). Regular physical activity is the third pillar: you needn't be an ironman triathlete; a brisk half-hour walk or any moderate activity you enjoy, done consistently, provides tremendous benefits for cardiovascular health, mood, and even creativity. If you're sedentary, moving into even a moderate activity routine can yield *outsized* improvements in fitness and reduce your risk of chronic disease dramatically. Additionally, avoiding destructive habits like smoking (or vaping) and heavy alcohol use has a huge pay-off in disease prevention – far more so than, say, taking the latest detox supplement or trying a charcoal cleanse.

To put it succinctly, master the basics first. They are the 20% of inputs giving you 80% of outcomes. Once your foundation is solid – you're sleeping adequately, moving regularly, eating mostly nourishing foods, and avoiding known health saboteurs – you will likely find you feel *so much better* that you're less tempted by gimmicks. Of course, everyone has individual preferences, so being a lazy genius also means personalizing what "matters" to you. Perhaps *meditation* is a small habit that yields big mental health benefits in your life; that could be part of your vital 20%. Or maybe you discover that drinking enough water and staying hydrated makes an outsized difference in your daily energy; then hydration is a key habit to prioritize. The strategy is to observe where you get the most bang-for-buck and allocate your effort accordingly.

Meanwhile, give yourself permission to be "lazy" about the wellness practices that don't matter as much. For instance, if you determine that fancy recovery supplements or elaborate skincare routines are not major contributors to your core health, feel free to simplify or ignore them. Many high-performing individuals actually thrive by simplifying choices – like eating a rotation of simple healthy meals and wearing a basic workout outfit – so they can direct their focus to truly important decisions. This is the lazy genius ethos: simplify the trivial to free up energy for the powerful. It's a form of efficiency in self-care. Notably, this approach is backed by behavior change science: trying to change too many things at once usually fails, whereas focusing on a few key behaviors is far more successful. By homing in on a short list of impactful habits, you avoid spreading yourself too thin or getting overwhelmed.

It may help to actually list out all the wellness "to-dos" swirling in your mind and then circle the few that genuinely give you the most benefit or joy. You might circle things like "go to bed by 10:30," "do a 20-min morning stretch routine," or "cook dinner at home 4 nights a week," depending on your life. Those are where you channel your inner genius – plan for them, protect time for them, even invest money in them if needed (for example, spending on good running shoes if running is your key habit). The rest of the list, you can allow yourself to do imperfectly or occasionally (or drop entirely) without guilt. Adopting this 20% focus is incredibly liberating for overachievers who've been fighting the urge to do *everything*. It validates that you're not failing if you aren't meditating, and journaling, and doing yoga and training for a 10K all at once. Instead, you're succeeding by intelligently picking your battles.

A case in point: *Priya*, a startup executive, was overwhelmed by her attempt to follow a "perfect" wellness routine. She tried to implement a complex morning regimen (oil pulling, green smoothie, 1-hour gym class, journaling, etc.) on top of long workdays. Not surprisingly, she couldn't keep up – most days she would hit snooze and then feel like a failure for skipping half those rituals. After learning about the lazy genius method, Priya re-evaluated which practices truly made her feel good. She realized that a solid night's sleep and a simple 15-minute yoga flow in the morning gave her more energy and mental clarity than the elaborate routine ever did. She decided those two habits were non-negotiable (20% that mattered). She also identified that preparing a healthy lunch to take to work kept her diet on track. Everything else – from trying every new supplement to aiming for 10,000 steps at all cost – she labelled as "niceto-have." The result: Priya felt less stressed and guilty, and her core habits became second nature. She joked that she was *"lazily"* doing far less than before, yet she felt healthier than ever because she was focusing on what counts.

In summary, the lazy genius philosophy applied to wellness is about strategic effort. By zeroing in on a handful of high-yield habits, you cut through the noise of wellness trends and avoid the burnout of trying to be perfect. This approach acknowledges that our time and willpower are limited resources – a wise person uses them where they'll make the biggest difference. In the end, you create a personalized "minimal effective dose" of wellness: the smallest routine that gives you robust health benefits. Everything beyond that is optional. Adopting this mindset can transform wellness from an overwhelming full-time job into an *integrated, efficient part of your life*. You'll know you're doing enough, and you can actually enjoy your life instead of constantly stressing about optimizing it.

Balance Beats Burnout

In a society that often glorifies the hustle – late-night grinds, early mornings, and the ethos of *"no pain, no gain"* – it's revolutionary to assert that rest and balance can actually fuel success better than endless work. Yet cutting-edge insights in neuroscience, physiology, and even corporate productivity are all coalescing around one truth: *humans are not machines*. We function best when we oscillate between periods of focused effort and periods of recovery. Sufficient rest, relaxation, and work-life balance are not signs of weakness or slacking; on the contrary, they are proven performance enhancers and protective factors against burnout. Embracing balance is an act of strength and wisdom – one that allows you to stay sane, replenish your energy, and ultimately achieve more in the long run.

Consider the science of rest and performance. A famous study by NASA found that when pilots took a short nap – just 26 minutes – during long flights, their alertness shot up by 54% and their job performance improved by 34% compared to pilots who didn't nap. In essence, a brief rest boosted their effectiveness by *one-third*. That's a striking statistic, and it underscores a broader point: adequate rest can boost productivity more than constant grinding. Other research consistently shows that well-rested individuals think more clearly, react faster, and solve problems more creatively. By contrast, when we push past our limits and skimp on rest, our cognitive resources get depleted. We've all experienced the foggy thinking or irritability that comes from too little sleep or no breaks during a hectic day. In fact, studies on work breaks find that *not* taking breaks leads to diminishing returns — attention and accuracy decline over time — whereas even short micro-breaks help maintain performance, especially on long tasks. Far from being time wasted, rest is time invested in sharper performance later. As one wellness report succinctly put it, "Rest is not the opposite of productivity; it's what sustains it".

Beyond momentary performance, adequate rest is integral to long-term health and preventing burnout. Burnout – characterized by chronic exhaustion, cynicism, and reduced efficacy – has become a rampant problem in modern work culture. The World Health Organization now recognizes burnout as an occupational phenomenon, closely tied to unrelenting stress without sufficient recovery. Simply put, if you never allow yourself to recharge, you eventually grind to a halt. Medical research draws a direct line between lack of rest and various health issues: chronic sleep deprivation and overwork are associated with increased risk of cardiovascular disease, suppressed immune function, insulin resistance, and mental health struggles like depression and anxiety. On the flip side, adequate rest improves emotional resilience and stability. When you're well-rested, you cope with challenges better and are less likely to be derailed by minor frustrations. One analysis even suggests that rest and leisure activities help replenish our mental resources and build resilience to stress – in other words, taking time off actually makes you *tougher* in the face of adversity because you're recharging your capacity to handle it.

Modern corporate experiments echo these findings. Trials of the four-day workweek in various companies have found that when employees work one day less (with the same pay), they often maintain or even *increase* productivity, while markers of well-being improve markedly. For instance, a six-month large-scale trial in the UK recently reported significant reductions in burnout and stress among employees who moved to a 32-hour workweek, alongside stable or higher company outputs. These real-world experiments challenge the old assumption that more hours = more output; instead, *working smarter with sufficient downtime yields better results.* Companies that encourage vacations, reasonable work hours, and respect for off-clock time often see lower turnover and higher engagement. It turns out humans operate best not under constant pressure, but when they have balance – much like an athlete who performs best when their training regimen *builds in* rest days and recovery periods.

Indeed, sports science provides a perfect parallel: elite athletes treat rest and recovery as equally important as training. Muscles actually strengthen and grow during rest, not during the workout itself (during exercise they experience micro-tears, and it's the subsequent rest period that allows them to repair stronger). Coaches of top Olympic teams enforce rest days, sleep hygiene, massage, and mental breaks, knowing that an overtrained athlete is prone to injury and decline in performance. The same principle applies to anyone striving in work or personal goals – pushing without pause is counterproductive. Adequate sleep, relaxation techniques, and downtime aren't indulgences; they are part of the formula for sustained high performance. In one memorable example, Google implemented nap pods and "20% time" (where employees could spend part of their week on creative projects or learning) and found it fueled innovation. Rest, it seems, feeds the very creativity and strategic thinking that intensive work alone cannot generate.

Perhaps the most persuasive voices on the importance of balance are those who learned the hard way. Media mogul Arianna Huffington famously experienced a wake-up call in 2007 when she *collapsed* in her office from exhaustion, hitting her head and breaking her cheekbone. Doctors told her the cause was extreme sleep deprivation and burnout. Reflecting on that incident later, Huffington realized she had bought into the false idol of hustling at the expense of health. She became a vocal advocate for sleep and balance. As she put it, "It's a delusion that in order to succeed as an entrepreneur you need to burn out." In fact, she noted that the greatest growth of her company happened *after* she started prioritizing sleep and well-being. Once she began getting 7–8 hours of sleep, she found herself more joyful, less reactive, and a better leader – able to make decisions with clarity rather than clouded by fatigue. Huffington highlights a cultural shift we need: recognizing that human beings are not machines. Whereas machines are optimized by minimizing downtime, humans are optimized by strategic downtime. "The goal of a machine is to minimize downtime, but human beings are not machines," she observed. "The need for eight hours' sleep is evolutionary, it's not negotiable. If we ignore that need, we pay a huge price in every aspect of our health and cognitive performance". Her words encapsulate the new paradigm: rest is a feature, not a bug, of a healthy and productive life.

To embrace balance as a strength, we should actively set boundaries and prioritize recovery in daily life. This might mean establishing a firm cutoff in the evenings beyond which work emails go unanswered, or committing to a regular relaxing activity (like reading, gentle stretching, or time with loved ones) that isn't "productive" in the traditional sense. It certainly means protecting your sleep as non-negotiable. If you have been sacrificing sleep for other goals, it may be the single most impactful change to reverse that habit. The research is unequivocal that good sleep enhances memory, mood, and even metabolic health, whereas chronic lack of sleep undermines them. Similarly, *taking breaks* during the day should be seen as responsible behavior, not laziness. A short walk outside or a calm cup of tea away from your desk can reset your concentration and prevent mental fatigue. One study found that longer breaks yielded greater boosts in performance, and even brief "micro-breaks" improved well-being without detracting from work goals. The key is intention: treat rest as a *skill* you cultivate, just like focus.

Finally, embracing balance involves a mindset shift: understanding that saying "no" or taking time off can be a form of strength. It's a way of preserving your most precious asset – your mental and physical health – so that you can continue to show up fully in your work and life. In practice, this could mean declining extra commitments when your plate is full, or taking a mental health day when you're nearing burnout, without guilt. Far from falling behind, you'll likely return to your tasks with renewed vigor and creativity. In the long run, a balanced approach beats burnout because it's *sustainable.* You're not sprinting until you collapse; you're running a marathon at a pace that you can maintain, with rest stations along the way. As the saying goes, "you can't pour from an empty cup." By refilling your cup regularly – through sleep, relaxation, hobbies, time with loved ones – you ensure that you have something to pour into your work, your family, and your passions for years to come.

Redefining wellness for real life means discarding the extremes and toxic definitions that have held us back. In this chapter, we challenged all-or-nothing thinking and saw that small consistent habits beat dramatic sporadic efforts. We reframed healthy living as an act of self-care – something you do *because you deserve to feel good*, not because you need to punish yourself. We applied the lazy genius lens to wellness, focusing on the few habits that truly matter and giving ourselves grace to let go of the rest. And we embraced balance and rest as integral components of success, rather than signs of weakness. Together, these perspectives form a saner, kinder, and more effective health philosophy. Life is too short (and too precious) to spend it on burnout, self-criticism, or chasing unrealistic ideals. By redefining wellness in these ways, we choose a path of sustainable vitality – one where we can get fit, stay sane, and actually enjoy our lives, all at the same time. This anti-hustle health plan isn't about doing less for its own sake; it's about doing *enough*, and doing it with joy and wisdom. In the chapters ahead, we'll continue building on these principles, exploring practical strategies to make wellness fit seamlessly into your busy, beautifully imperfect real life. Because true wellness isn't a ruthless sprint; it's a gentle dance of consistent steps, self-compassion, focused effort, and rejuvenating rest – a dance that anyone, even the busiest or most burnt-out among us, can learn to enjoy.

Chapter 3

Mind-Body Reset – Stress and Mental Wellness

The Stress Effect: Hustle Culture's Toll on Body and Mind

Hustle culture glorifies being busy – the endless grind, long hours, and always being "on." Yet this relentless pursuit of success comes at a high cost to our health. Chronic stress becomes a lifestyle rather than a warning sign. When we live in a constant state of urgency, our bodies stay stuck in fight-or-flight mode. Stress hormones like cortisol surge and rarely get a chance to shut off. Over time, this hormonal overdrive wreaks havoc on both body and mind. Prolonged elevated cortisol disrupts nearly every system in the body, contributing to anxiety, depression, digestive issues, tension headaches, high blood pressure, and even weight gain. In fact, the World Health Organization found that consistently working over 55 hours per week dramatically raises the risk of heart disease and stroke. It's as if we're driving a car full speed on fumes – expecting peak performance while our tank is empty. The result is often brain fog, irritability, and exhaustion, even if we're ostensibly "achieving" more. Ironically, all that hustle can undercut our fitness gains and wellness goals: high cortisol makes it harder to build muscle, easier to accumulate fat, and leaves us too drained to exercise or make healthy choices.

Chronic overwork and stress can leave us feeling physically exhausted and mentally drained, like a car running on empty. In hustle culture, being "busy" becomes a badge of honor even as our bodies and minds begin to falter.

Living in a perpetual stress response also frays our mental resilience. Small problems start to feel like crises when your nervous system never gets a break. You might notice you're anxious all the time or quick to anger. Concentration and creativity plummet due to mental fatigue. Sleep often suffers – either you can't fall asleep with your mind racing, or you wake up at 3 AM thinking about emails. This creates a vicious cycle: poor sleep increases stress, and more stress further wrecks sleep. Over time, chronic stress can lead to burnout, a state of total mental and physical exhaustion. Burnout isn't just feeling a bit tired – it's characterized by cynicism, detachment, and a sense of ineffectiveness. Your passion and motivation evaporate. Alarming surveys show up to three-quarters of people worldwide report struggling with burnout in recent years. In other words, feeling perpetually stressed and overwhelmed has practically become the norm. But it *is* possible to break out of this cycle. First, we need to recognize the red flags of burnout before we hit a breaking point.

Breaking the Burnout Cycle: From Breakdown to Breakthrough

Meet Jason, a 38-year-old marketing director and classic overachiever. For years, Jason routinely clocked 70-hour workweeks, prided himself on being the first in and last out of the office, and answered emails at midnight. He told himself this grind was necessary to succeed. But gradually, the cracks began to show. He became easily agitated over minor issues at work. At home, he was physically present but mentally distant – too fatigued to play with his kids and skipping family dinners to catch up on work. Sleep eluded him; he'd jolt awake with his heart pounding, thinking about quarterly targets. One morning before a big client meeting, Jason experienced chest pains and dizziness. It was his wake-up call. At the doctor's office, he was warned that his blood pressure was dangerously high and that he was on the verge of burnout-induced collapse. Jason finally had to confront the reality: if he didn't change his approach, his hustle was going to hurt him more than it helped him.

Jason's story is a composite of countless real-world professionals who hit a wall from chronic overwork. The good news is that burnout can be addressed before it reaches a crisis. The first step is learning to recognize the warning signs. Common signs include feeling drained every morning, loss of motivation or joy in work you once loved, increased cynicism or irritability, and declines in performance. Often, you stop taking care of yourself – skipping workouts, eating poorly, neglecting sleep. You might withdraw from friends or family because you're "too busy" or simply don't have the energy. When work starts to consume your identity and all your time, it's a signal that something's off balance.

Breaking out of the burnout cycle means giving yourself *permission to pause*. This can feel counterintuitive to overachievers, but strategically stepping back is essential to moving forward. Start by injecting small breaks into your day. Research shows that even a five-minute walk outside or a few deep, deliberate breaths can reset your stress response and restore focus. Think of these micro-breaks as hitting the "refresh" button on your brain. For Jason, this meant actually taking a lunch break away from his desk (something he hadn't done in years) and doing short guided breathing exercises between meetings. At first, he felt guilty – as if he was slacking off. But he soon realized these pauses made him more productive in the afternoons and far calmer in the evenings.

Another key to interrupting burnout is setting realistic goals and boundaries. High achievers often fall into the trap of perfectionism, setting impossibly high standards for themselves. Jason reflected on how he used to stay at the office polishing a presentation that was 99% great, chasing that last 1% of "perfection" while his personal life suffered. He learned to reframe his mindset to "progress over perfection." This meant breaking projects into smaller, achievable steps and defining what "good enough" looked like for each step. Psychology experts note that celebrating small wins triggers dopamine hits in the brain, reinforcing motivation and momentum. In practice, Jason began acknowledging each task completed (rather than fixating on everything left undone) and set explicit "stop times" for work in the evening. He also communicated with his team about priorities, so he didn't feel solely responsible for every outcome.

Equally important, Jason started to seek support instead of silently soldiering on. He opened up to a close colleague about feeling burnt out, and discovered she and others felt the same way. Together they approached their manager about more reasonable deadline setting and cross-training team members to share the load. He also talked with his family, apologizing for his absence and enlisting their encouragement to stick to his new boundaries. Whether it's talking to a friend, a partner, a mentor, or a therapist, getting support can be a lifesaver. Burnout often carries a sense of isolation – the feeling that it's all on you – but that's an illusion. Simply verbalizing your stress can relieve some of its power, and others can help you brainstorm solutions or at least remind you that you're not alone.

Over time, these changes pulled Jason out of his downward spiral. By catching burnout early and making modest shifts – a walk here, an honest conversation there, a line drawn between work and home – he interrupted the pattern before it became a full collapse. The takeaway: you don't need to quit your job or take a six-month sabbatical to break the burnout cycle (though in some cases, a vacation or leave can help). Small, consistent steps make a tangible difference. As one burnout coach puts it, *"Boundaries and breaks are not laziness; they're your lifelines."* Realistically adjust your workload, build recovery into your routine, and don't wait for a crisis to make a change. By doing so, you can restore your energy and passion *before* it's too late.

Mindfulness and Mental Resilience: Stress Reduction in Seconds a Day

One of the most powerful antidotes to stress and burnout is literally right under our noses – our breath. Mindfulness meditation and relaxation techniques have moved from monasteries into the mainstream for good reason: *they work*. You don't have to retreat to a mountaintop or commit to an hour of yoga daily to reap the benefits, either. Even a few minutes of mindfulness practiced consistently can significantly reduce stress and anxiety. In fact, researchers reviewing over 200 studies of mindfulness found that mindfulness-based therapy is especially effective for lowering stress, anxiety, and depression. When you're mindful, you train your brain to focus on the present moment rather than ruminating about past regrets or future worries – and this mental shift has measurable effects on the body. Studies show that regular mindfulness practice can lower cortisol levels in chronically stressed individuals, improving everything from blood pressure to immune function.

Perhaps even more impressive, mindfulness helps tame emotional reactivity, including anger. If you've ever felt on a hair-trigger when stressed – snapping at a loved one or sending a fiery email you later regret – mindfulness can build the pause button into your responses. A recent meta-analysis of 118 studies found that people who learned mindfulness skills demonstrated *less anger and aggressive behavior* in their lives. In other words, practicing mindfulness can make you less likely to explode in an angry outburst and more likely to respond calmly, even under pressure. It's not magic or mysticism; it's the result of training your mind to observe feelings without immediately reacting. Over time, you strengthen the mental muscle that lets you notice "I'm getting upset" and choose a wiser response. Many participants in these studies ranged from busy professionals to students, showing that the benefits of mindfulness are broadly accessible and universal.

Importantly, mindfulness and relaxation techniques can fit into the busiest schedule – they are truly tools for "lazy geniuses" who want maximum benefit in minimum time. The key is consistency and finding practices that resonate with you. Here are a few simple, science-backed exercises you can try right away:

- **The One-Minute Breath Break:** Sit comfortably, soften your gaze or close your eyes, and take slow deep breaths for 60 seconds. Inhale through your nose for a count of 4, let your belly expand. Exhale through your mouth for a count of 6 or 8, allowing tension to release. If your mind wanders (and it will), gently bring your focus back to the breath. Even one minute of conscious breathing can lower your heart rate and calm your nerves. Busy executives have used this technique before high-stakes meetings to great effect – it's a quick reset for your racing mind.

- **Body Scan for Busy People:** While lying down to sleep or even sitting at your desk, take 2-3 minutes to mentally scan your body from head to toe. Notice any areas of tightness (tense shoulders, clenched jaw) and consciously invite those muscles to relax. This practice, often used in mindfulness-based stress reduction (MBSR), helps shift your focus out of a whirlwind mind into the calm of the body. It's been shown to reduce anxiety and improve sleep when done regularly.

- **Mindful Micro-Activity:** Turn a routine daily activity into a mindfulness session by giving it your full attention. For example, while drinking your morning coffee or tea, really notice the aroma, the warmth of the mug in your hand, and the taste with each sip. If thoughts about the day ahead intrude, acknowledge them and gently return to the sensory experience. This grounding in the present can prevent your brain from leaping straight into stress mode each morning. Some people find a mindful walk (even just from the parking lot to the office, noticing the feel of the ground and the air on your skin) has a similar calming effect.

By integrating these small practices, you're essentially training resilience. Mindfulness teaches your brain and body how to recover from stress more quickly. Many high-pressure companies have caught on – from Google to Goldman Sachs, mindfulness and meditation programs are offered to employees as tools to enhance focus and manage stress. A software engineer who tried his firm's 5-minute meditation session at lunch was surprised to find that his usual afternoon slump and temper flares diminished. "It's like I hit reset at midday," he said, "I come back to my desk feeling strangely recharged." You can do the same. Whether through an app-guided meditation in your car before driving home, a yoga class, or quiet moments in the shower focusing on the water hitting your skin, relaxation techniques are versatile and portable. The science is clear that these practices aren't indulgences – they're effective methods to protect your mental wellness amidst the chaos of a packed schedule. Over time, you may even find that mindfulness becomes a habit as routine as brushing your teeth, and its benefits – lower stress, steadier emotions, and a stronger mind-body connection – will only grow.

Reframing Your Inner Dialogue: The Mental Shifts of Resilience

While external practices like breaks and meditation are crucial, an often overlooked aspect of stress management is the conversation happening inside your own head. Our inner dialogue – the automatic thoughts and self-talk that run through our minds – can either amplify stress or help buffer it. In the hustle mindset, many of us have internal monologues that are harsh, critical, and perfectionistic. We push ourselves with thoughts like "I'm not doing enough," "I can't mess up," or "If I slow down, I'll fall behind." This mental chatter creates a constant background of pressure. To reset our mind-body balance, we must reframe that inner dialogue toward encouragement, compassion, and perspective. Science backs this up: individuals who practice positive self-talk and cultivate self-compassion experience significantly lower levels of distress and burnout.

One powerful reframing tool is gratitude. This isn't about forced positivity or pretending everything is perfect – it's about intentionally shifting focus to the good, even when stress is present. Studies have shown that people who regularly reflect on things they're grateful for have markedly lower cortisol levels and better ability to handle stress. In one study, participants who kept a daily gratitude journal (simply writing down a few things they appreciated each day) not only felt emotionally better, but their physical stress markers improved – they slept better and even had improved cardiac health. Gratitude works because it gently pulls your mind away from endless worry or negativity and reminds you of the resources and positives in your life. For a busy person, a simple practice is to take 30 seconds at the end of each day to mentally name three things that went well or brought joy. They can be as small as "had a delicious sandwich for lunch" or "my colleague helped me solve a problem." Over time, this trains your brain to notice positives more automatically, creating an emotional buffer against daily stress. As Dr. Kristin Francis of the Huntsman Mental Health Institute notes, expressing gratitude boosts serotonin and dopamine in the brain — neurotransmitters that make you feel good and help you bounce back from adversity. In essence, gratitude is a natural anti-depressant and anti-anxiety practice you can do anywhere, anytime.

Another crucial mindset shift is developing positive and realistic self-talk. When a setback happens, notice the tone of your inner voice. Do you berate yourself ("You always screw things up")? That kind of negative self-talk magnifies stress and erodes confidence. Now imagine reframing those thoughts as if you were speaking to a dear friend. You'd probably be more understanding: "This was a tough situation and you did your best," or "Mistakes happen — what can we learn and improve for next time?" This isn't just feel-good advice; optimism and positive self-talk have been linked to better coping and even physical health benefits. People with an optimistic explanatory style tend to see challenges as temporary and specific, rather than permanent personal failures. As a result, they experience lower levels of distress and better overall well-being. You can cultivate this by practicing what psychologists call cognitive reframing. For example, instead of "I have to do everything perfectly or I'll be a failure," reframe to "I want to do well, but I'm also allowed to be human. A mistake is not the end of the world." Over time, these gentler messages reduce the pressure cooker in your mind.

Perhaps the most profound inner shift is embracing self-compassion. This concept, championed by researchers like Dr. Kristin Neff, means treating yourself with the same kindness and understanding you'd offer to a friend. High achievers and busy people often have the opposite habit: self-criticism. But research shows that self-compassion is a secret weapon against burnout. In fact, a large body of studies finds that higher self-compassion correlates with significantly lower burnout, stress, and psychological distress. When you're self-compassionate, you acknowledge that you're struggling and offer yourself support rather than blame. For instance, instead of, "I should be stronger, I shouldn't be stressed by this," a self-compassionate approach says, "I'm really having a hard time right now, and that's okay – many people would feel this way in my shoes. What do I need to care for myself?" This mindset doesn't make you complacent; it actually builds resilience. By not wasting energy on self-blame, you can channel it into solutions and healing. One emergency room nurse shared that learning self-compassion techniques (like placing a hand on her heart and speaking to herself kindly during tough shifts) helped her recover from work stress much faster. Instead of spiraling into "What's wrong with me that I can't handle this?", she began telling herself, "This *is* really hard, and I'm doing my best. I deserve a break tonight." She found her anxiety decreased and her passion for her job returned once she stopped mentally beating herself up.

To start reframing your inner dialogue, you can use practical exercises. Try writing a letter to yourself from the perspective of a wise, compassionate friend – what would they say about your efforts and worth? Or practice a quick self-compassion break: when stress hits, pause and say to yourself, "This is a moment of stress. Stress is a part of life. May I give myself kindness in this moment." It might feel awkward at first, but these practices are proven to shift your mindset toward one of encouragement and patience. Remember, your mind believes what you tell it repeatedly. If you change the narrative from "not enough" to "doing my best," from "I must hustle" to "I must also heal," your body will follow by dialing down the stress response. Reframing inner dialogue is the ultimate "anti-hustle" mental tool – it allows you to stay ambitious and driven *without* destroying yourself in the process. By cultivating gratitude, positive self-talk, and self-compassion, you build an unshakable mental resilience. Instead of your mind being your biggest critic and source of stress, it becomes your greatest ally in living a healthy, sane, and genuinely enjoyable life. And that is the true genius of the "lazy wellness" approach: achieving more by *pushing less*, and caring for your mind as attentively as you care for your body.

Chapter 4

Movement That Fits Your Life

"Not everything that counts can be counted." This famous saying holds true for fitness. In a world that glorifies intense 5 a.m. workouts and grueling gym sessions, it's easy to believe that only the *hardcore* stuff "counts" as exercise. But guess what? Movement is movement – and all those little actions you take in a day truly add up. For busy professionals and burnt-out overachievers, embracing this idea can be life-changing. In this chapter, we'll explore how to fit movement into your life *on your terms*. You'll learn why everyday activities matter for your health, how to rediscover exercise as play, ways to overcome "gym dread," and the big benefits of tiny workouts. The goal is to break free from all-or-nothing thinking and find a sustainable, enjoyable approach to staying active. Let's dive in with some grounded science, real-world examples, and a dose of motivational wisdom.

Everyday Activity Counts: The Power of NEAT

For years, many of us have equated "exercise" with scheduled sweat sessions – a spin class here, a CrossFit WOD there. But what about the other 23 hours of your day? The truth is that all the *everyday* movements you do (or don't do) have a profound impact on your health. Scientists even have a name for it: Non-Exercise Activity Thermogenesis, thankfully nicknamed NEAT, which is the energy you burn through everything that's not formal exercise – literally "everything we do that is not sleeping, eating or sports-like exercise." This includes walking to your car, pacing during a phone call, cleaning the house, chasing your toddler, or even fidgeting in a meeting. It might not sound like much, but every bit counts. Over time, these little movements can add up to significant benefits.

Just how powerful is NEAT? Research shows there's a *huge* variability between individuals in how many calories they burn via daily activity. In fact, NEAT can differ by up to 2,000 calories per day between two people of similar size. That's the difference between someone who's sedentary (think: desk job, drives everywhere, watches TV at night) and someone who's naturally active in daily life (perhaps they stand, walk, putter around and rarely sit still). In other words, *habits matter.* If you've ever wondered why a friend stays slim without ever hitting the gym, NEAT may be the answer. Those extra calories burned by taking the stairs, doing yardwork, or restless fidgeting can significantly impact weight management. As one review notes, targeting NEAT – simply moving more in daily life – can be a crucial tool for controlling body weight.

But weight is only one part of the story. The health benefits of everyday activity go well beyond burning calories. When you integrate more movement into your routine – standing up regularly, walking, cleaning, gardening, you name it – you're protecting your body from the harms of being too sedentary. Studies have found that people who move more and sit less tend to have better heart health, circulation, and blood sugar levels, experience fewer aches and pains, and even report improved focus, mood, and energy. It makes sense: our bodies evolved to move, not to be hunched over a laptop all day. Even small actions can stimulate your muscles and blood flow, triggering the release of feel-good brain chemicals and boosting your mental clarity. Ever notice how a quick walk around the block can lift your mood during an afternoon slump? That's NEAT in action, improving your day in subtle but meaningful ways.

Crucially, these everyday movements all contribute to your fitness – even if they don't look anything like a traditional workout. One fascinating study showed that even a single "brisk minute" of moving – say, a quick climb up the office stairs or a burst of energetic housecleaning – had a measurable impact on health. Women who peppered their days with short bursts of activity had slightly lower BMI and lower odds of obesity than those who remained entirely sedentary. "Every movement counts" isn't just a slogan; it's scientific fact. Over time, the calories burned and the cardiovascular boosts from these mini-movements can significantly improve your overall fitness and quality of life.

If you're thinking *"Sure, but I still need real exercise eventually,"* you're not wrong – dedicated exercise has its own benefits. But reframing your mindset to value everyday activity is liberating. It frees you from the unhealthy notion that *only* a 60-minute cardio class or a hardcore gym session is worthwhile. Vacuuming the living room or walking the dog may not feel like exercise, but they absolutely contribute to your health. In fact, look at communities known for longevity: in the famous "Blue Zones" (regions where people routinely live into their 90s and 100s in good health), folks don't hit the gym at all. Instead, they "stay active through daily, natural movements like gardening, walking, and manual housework," seamlessly integrating activity into life. The result? Long, healthy lives. The lesson for us is clear – you don't have to grind out formal workouts to reap benefits. Parking farther from the store, taking the stairs, doing a little dance while cooking dinner, playing with your kids or pets – it all matters. These micro-movements keep your body from prolonged stillness (which we know is harmful) and create a foundation of health.

One key concept here is to break up long periods of sitting. Health experts warn that "oversitting" (sitting for hours at a time) can lead to metabolic issues like high blood pressure, elevated blood sugar, and high cholesterol. If you have a desk job, make it a point to stand up or stroll regularly. Set a timer to remind yourself to stretch or walk for a couple of minutes each hour. Not only will this burn a few extra calories, but you'll likely return to your task with a clearer mind and more energy. NEAT, in effect, helps counteract the modern sedentary lifestyle that saps our vitality. As Dr. Anas Dakkak of the Cleveland Clinic puts it, even though NEAT alone won't magically make you lose 10 pounds overnight, it's an "opportunity to make small but meaningful changes" that give your body an edge. Those edges add up. Over weeks and months, you might notice you feel a bit stronger carrying groceries, less stiff after long drives, or more upbeat during the workday thanks to the extra movement.

So, *take heart*: every day is filled with chances to move more, without needing any special gear or dedicated time slot. It could be as simple as standing up to take phone calls, doing calf raises while you brush your teeth, or enthusiastically scrubbing the bathtub (yes, housework counts!). Think of these not as chores, but as stealth exercise. By embracing NEAT and valuing everyday activity, you're building a lifestyle where movement happens naturally. You're treating your body to what it craves – frequent motion – and freeing yourself from the "all or nothing" gym mindset. In sum, tiny lifestyle tweaks can yield big health rewards.

Exercise Reimagined as Play: Finding Joy in Movement

If the word "exercise" conjures images of slogging on a treadmill or punishing yourself with burpees, it's time for a mental reset. Movement can be *fun*. In fact, to make exercise a sustainable habit, it should be fun (or at least enjoyable in some way). Let's banish the notion that fitness has to feel like self-inflicted torture. Instead, we'll reimagine exercise as play – as something you genuinely look forward to. Whether it's dancing in your living room, hiking to a beautiful viewpoint, roller skating, or playing pickleball with friends, finding activities you enjoy is the magic ingredient to staying active long-term. Science backs this up: *enjoyment* isn't a luxury here, it's a necessity for consistency and success.

Consider the last time you did something active that made you laugh or smile. Maybe you had an impromptu dance party to your favorite song and ended up breathless with a grin on your face. Or you joined a casual sports league (kickball, anyone?) and realized an hour flew by without you checking the clock once. That feeling of losing yourself in an activity is what we're after. When exercise feels like play, it stops being a chore on your to-do list and becomes something you want to do. Researchers have found that enjoyment is a powerful predictor of whether people stick with physical activity. In one study, exercise enjoyment turned out to be a better predictor of long-term persistence than even "motivation" or external goals like weight loss. In other words, you might start exercising because you *think you should* (to get healthier, to lose weight, etc.), but you'll only keep doing it if you're getting some genuine pleasure or satisfaction from it. As one report succinctly put it, "enjoyment [is] the main reason for exercisers to participate in sports activities over the long term" – it motivates and anchors their adherence.

This makes perfect sense. Think about hobbies you stick with – maybe a musical instrument, gardening, or playing chess. You do them because they light you up, not because someone is holding you accountable. Why should exercise be any different? It turns out that even among people with serious health concerns, *fun* is a deciding factor. A U.S. study of patients with heart failure found that even though these individuals were highly motivated to improve their health, they were less likely to exercise if they didn't enjoy the activity. That's striking – even life-or-death stakes weren't as effective in prompting exercise as the simple factor of enjoyment. As Dr. Matthew Bourke, a movement researcher, explains, "If you look forward to it, you're going to keep doing it."

So how do you find the joy in movement if you've long associated exercise with drudgery or embarrassment? Start by rethinking what counts as exercise. There are no rules that say you must run on a treadmill or lift weights in a gym for it to be legitimate. Maybe you love music – try a Zumba class, a dance-based video game, or just crank up tunes at home and dance like nobody's watching. Maybe you're competitive – join a recreational sports league or challenge a friend to weekly tennis matches. Maybe you crave nature and solitude – go hiking, trail running, or biking in the park. Or perhaps you miss the carefree play of childhood – you could try rollerblading, hula hooping, or even an adult trampoline class (yes, those exist!). One person struggling with fitness discovered an "intro to pole dancing" class and found it was actually really fun, as shared on an anti-diet forum – it became a form of exercise she eagerly attended, because it felt playful and empowering rather than like punishment.

Remember, the *best* exercise is the one you'll actually do. If you genuinely hate something, it's unlikely you'll stick with it long enough to see results. On the other hand, if an activity makes you happy (or at least leaves you feeling good afterward), you'll naturally want to do it more often – and *that* consistency brings results over time. The latest science confirms this: studies show that people who find physical activities they enjoy have higher exercise adherence and better long-term outcomes. Enjoyment even seems to amplify the benefits – Dr. Bourke notes that while any exercise has mental and physical benefits, "more enjoyment does bring more gains" in the long run. When you're engaged and having fun, you might push a bit harder or stay active a bit longer without even realizing it, compared to forcing yourself through a joyless routine while watching the clock.

Let's put this into a real-world perspective. Think of two people, Alice and Bob. Alice forces herself to do a popular high-intensity interval class because she heard it burns lots of calories, but she secretly despises every minute – it's too intense, the music annoys her, and she feels self-conscious. Bob, on the other hand, loves biking, so he starts going on evening bike rides with a couple of friends from work, exploring different neighborhoods and grabbing a smoothie afterward. A month later, who's more likely to have stuck with their exercise routine? Bob – because he's genuinely enjoying it. Alice skips one class, then another, and soon "falls off the wagon," reinforcing her belief that she's lazy or bad at exercising. The moral: find your "bike rides with friends," whatever form that takes. It could be joining a weekly walking group so you can chat as you move, or signing up for a beginner-friendly yoga class that doubles as stress relief, or turning your daily dog walk into an adventure by exploring new routes. Exercise doesn't have to look traditional to count. As long as you're moving and it makes you feel good, it's valid.

If you're not sure what you enjoy, treat it like an experiment. Make a list of physical activities that *sound* appealing or that you enjoyed in the past (did you love swimming as a kid? dancing at parties? playing basketball in school?). Then try them out! Give yourself permission to be a beginner and to have fun with it. When you hit on something that leaves you smiling and pleasantly tired, you've struck gold. Over time, these "playful" exercises can get you just as fit as any structured workout plan. In fact, you might find you go longer or harder in a fun activity without noticing, whereas 10 minutes on a treadmill feels like an eternity. One systematic review even noted that people often report higher enjoyment (and no loss of effectiveness) with varied, high-intensity interval training compared to monotonous steady exercise. The bottom line is that enjoyment has the greatest impact on exercise persistence. So go ahead and prioritize fun. It's not frivolous – it's the key to making movement a lifelong habit. As one fitness writer put it, "We make exercise too complicated, but it doesn't have to be… rather than seeing exercise as a chore, we can use it as a tool to feel better" – keep it simple and enjoyable.

Overcoming Gym Aversion: Finding Your Comfort Zone

If the mere thought of entering a gym makes you anxious – the glaring mirrors, the clanking machines, the crowds of people who all seem to know what they're doing – you're *far* from alone. "Gym intimidation" (cheekily dubbed "gymtimidation") is a real phenomenon. Many people, especially those just starting out or restarting their fitness journey, feel self-conscious and out of place in typical gym environments. Common fears include: *"Everyone will stare at me and judge me," "I don't know how to use these machines, I'll embarrass myself,"* or *"I don't look fit enough to be here."* These worries can be paralyzing – in one survey, many women reported avoiding the weight room despite knowing the benefits of strength training, mainly because they feared being perceived as uncoordinated or out of place. The result is that a space meant for health ends up feeling exclusionary. So let's address this head on: you do not have to go to a gym to be active. If you hate the gym, there are *plenty* of other ways to get moving that might suit you better. And if you *want* to use the gym but feel nervous, there are strategies to make it more comfortable. Let's tackle both angles.

Option 1: Skip the gym – you have alternatives. Some people truly thrive in a gym setting, but many do not. And that's okay! There is nothing magical about those four walls. The key is finding an environment where you feel comfortable and motivated to move. Here are some creative alternatives:

- **Work Out at Home:** With today's technology, you can get a great workout in your living room or bedroom. There are countless fitness apps and free YouTube videos offering everything from yoga and Pilates to kickboxing and dance cardio. Even if you have no equipment, you'll find bodyweight routines that get your heart rate up. Home workouts have boomed in popularity – during the 2020 pandemic lockdowns, Google searches for "home workouts" spiked by 78% as people sought ways to stay active indoors. Many discovered that exercising at home is convenient (no commute, no packing a gym bag) and *private* (no worry about how you look or what others think). Busy professional on Zoom calls all day? You can squeeze in short exercise breaks (more on "exercise snacks" soon) or do a quick 20-minute video in the morning before you shower. Over time, a consistent home workout routine can absolutely get you in shape. Some of the fittest folks on Instagram are using just a mat and resistance bands at home. The key is consistency and finding online instructors or programs you enjoy so that pressing "Play" feels inviting, not like drudgery.

- **Get Outdoors:** There's a whole world outside the gym waiting for you. Maybe the idea of running on a treadmill makes you cringe, but jogging through a park or along a river sounds much nicer. Fresh air and scenery can make a huge difference in your exercise experience. You could start with brisk walks in your neighborhood and gradually incorporate short jogging intervals – many people have had success with programs like Couch to 5K using this gentle approach. If running's not your thing, consider cycling – either outdoors or on a bike share – or simply long walks/hikes on local trails. Even a casual bike ride or walk will get your blood flowing. Other ideas: join a local sports league (soccer, softball, ultimate Frisbee – the emphasis is on fun at the recreational level), try outdoor swimming at a community pool or lake, or find a nearby tennis or basketball court and shoot some hoops for fun. The bonus? Exercising in nature can boost mood *extra* effectively. Studies suggest that being outdoors amplifies the cognitive and psychological benefits of physical activity. Sunlight, trees, and a breeze can be incredibly refreshing after a day at a desk. And outside, there's no one monitoring your "performance" – no mirrors, no judgy vibes. It's just you and your environment.

- **Find a Friendly Tribe:** Sometimes the issue isn't exercise itself but feeling alone or unsupported. Maybe you actually do better with some social motivation – just not in the intimidating gym context. In that case, look for more welcoming movement communities. This could be a group fitness class geared toward beginners or a specific demographic (there are classes for seniors, postpartum moms, larger-bodied folks, etc., which may feel more inclusive). It might be a dance studio that fosters a body-positive environment, or a small bootcamp group in a park where everyone is friendly and encouraging. A great example is the rise of walking groups and community run clubs that explicitly welcome all paces – you might find a weekly walking meetup where the focus is on chatting and enjoyment, not speed. If the first group or class you try doesn't feel like a fit, try another. When you find *your people* – those who cheer for you and make exercise fun – it can transform your attitude toward working out. Suddenly it's not "I have to exercise," but "I get to go play and see my friends." As an added benefit, having a workout buddy or group can help with accountability on days your motivation wanes.

- **Different Gym Vibe:** If you *do* want the equipment or resources of a gym, remember that not all gyms are alike. A massive, packed commercial gym might not feel great if you're anxious, but how about a smaller boutique gym or a women-only gym or a YMCA? Some gyms pride themselves on being extra welcoming to newbies. "A smaller, more inclusive gym may help you conquer your gym anxiety," notes one fitness expert. These environments might have more approachable staff, a less macho atmosphere, or a community feel. You could also consider scheduling an orientation with a trainer so you learn the basics when the gym is quieter, or go during off-peak hours initially (e.g. mid-afternoon rather than the 6 p.m. rush). Over time, as you become familiar with the layout and equipment, your confidence will grow. Remember, everyone at the gym was a beginner at some point – truly, *everyone*. Those fit-looking folks weren't born knowing how to use the squat rack; they had to learn too. And most people are far more focused on their own workout (or their own insecurities) to pay much attention to others. It can help to reframe your thinking: rather than "I don't belong here," tell yourself "I have as much right as anyone to use this space for my well-being". Because you absolutely do. Your health matters more than any imagined judgment.

Ultimately, the dread factor is what we want to remove. If you find yourself consistently dreading a particular workout setting, change it. Life is too short and health is too important to torture yourself with a mode of exercise or a venue you hate. As one mental health-oriented fitness guide put it, *anything that gets your body moving and your heart pumping can count as exercise*. That might be dancing in your kitchen, doing Pilates in your pajamas, hiking a trail, or yes, lifting weights at the gym – it's your call. There is no one-size-fits-all. By finding the right environment, you set yourself up for success because you remove a huge barrier. Instead of battling anxiety or boredom, you can focus on the joy and benefits of movement.

A quick case study: Janelle, a 35-year-old marketing executive, used to sign up for fancy gym memberships every New Year – and by March, she'd stop going. "I finally admitted to myself I just hate the gym," she says. Crowds and complicated machines stressed her out, and she felt guilty for not using the membership. So Janelle tried something new: she canceled the gym and invested in a good pair of walking shoes and some basic home equipment (a yoga mat and a few resistance bands). Each morning, instead of driving to the gym, she walked her dog for 30 minutes in the neighborhood, often inviting a friend or listening to her favorite podcast. At lunch, she did a 15-minute YouTube strength routine at home. The result? "It's been over a year, and I've actually stuck with it," Janelle reports. She's fitter and, more importantly, far less stressed. She looks forward to her walks as a time to clear her head. By removing the dread factor, she made movement a pleasant part of her daily life rather than a torture session she'd inevitably avoid.

The takeaway here is one of empowerment: *you* are in charge of your fitness journey. If the traditional gym route gives you the heebie-jeebies, you have permission to forge a different path. What matters is that you're moving regularly in ways that you can sustain. Find your comfort zone, whether that's a living room, a hiking trail, a dance floor, or a judgment-free gym where you feel at home. When you feel comfortable, you're far more likely to stay consistent – and consistency is the secret sauce of fitness.

Tiny Workouts, Big Benefits: "Exercise Snacks" for Busy Days

One of the most exciting insights in exercise science in recent years is the validation that short bursts of activity – even just a few minutes at a time – can deliver significant health benefits. This is a game-changer for busy people (and who isn't busy these days?). No matter how packed your schedule, you can squeeze in these "bite-sized" workouts, often called "exercise snacks." Just like you might grab a quick snack to keep your energy up between meals, you can do quick bouts of movement between bouts of sitting. The research is compelling: multiple mini-workouts spread through the day might even outperform a single longer workout when it comes to certain health metrics, especially if that longer workout is followed by hours of sitting. The key is consistency – doing these little bursts regularly.

So, what exactly is an exercise snack? Think of 30 seconds to 5 minutes of activity at a time. It could be as vigorous as climbing a few flights of stairs or as gentle as doing some yoga stretches at your desk, depending on your ability and context. The concept, as described by Dr. Marily Oppezzo of Stanford, is to fit in short bouts of movement that "get your heart rate up to a vigorous level" without requiring a trip to the gym or a change of clothes. For example, if you have a minute or two, you might jog in place or do jumping jacks until you're slightly out of breath. If high-intensity isn't your style, even a brisk walk around the building or some fast-paced stair climbing counts. These mini-workouts can be sprinkled through your day – morning, lunch break, between meetings, whenever. Over the course of a day, they accumulate into a meaningful amount of exercise.

Let's talk benefits, because they are truly *outsize* relative to the time investment. Research shows that performing short "exercise snacks" throughout the day can lead to improvements in cardiorespiratory fitness, endurance, and even muscle strength. One recent study found that just three 1-2 minute bursts of intense activity, done three times a day (so around 6 minutes total), seven days a week, significantly improved cardiovascular health in participants. Another study in sedentary individuals showed that brief stair-climbing snacks (three 20-second all-out climbs spread out in a day) increased fitness by about 5% over six weeks – not too shabby for such a tiny time commitment. The cumulative effect of these short bouts is comparable to traditional workouts in some respects. And importantly, they help break up long periods of sitting, which, as we discussed, is crucial for metabolic health.

Even beyond formal studies, the evidence is in our daily lives. Think about those days when you barely move versus days when you intersperse activity: if you spend a whole day sitting in marathon meetings, you probably feel achy and drained by evening. But if you take a few *activity breaks* – maybe you step outside for a 10-minute walk at lunch, do a quick stretch mid-afternoon, and play with your kids or pets after work – you likely end the day feeling more energized and in a better mood. There's a reason some offices now encourage "movement breaks" and provide standing desks or even under-desk ellipticals. Movement, even short, boosts our energy and alertness. One neuroscientist described it vividly:

every time you exercise, your brain is "taking a bubble bath" of neurochemical goodness. You come back refreshed.

To implement exercise snacks, it helps to attach them to existing routines. For instance, take the stairs instead of the elevator whenever possible – and if you have a couple extra minutes, go *up and down* an extra time or two for good measure (instant heart rate boost!). If you work on a certain floor, you could make it a habit to use a restroom on a different floor so you have to take the stairs. Or consider walking meetings: instead of sitting in a conference room, suggest walking with your colleague while you discuss. Not only will you get steps in, but walking can spur creativity. Some companies have embraced this, holding meetings on the move, which has the side benefit of often making discussions more lively and efficient

Here are a few "exercise snack" ideas to incorporate into your day-to-day life:

- **Morning stretch and strength:** Upon waking or before you dive into work, spend 5 minutes on a quick routine. For example: 10 bodyweight squats, 10 push-ups (can be against a wall or desk if needed), and a few minutes of stretching (roll your shoulders, twist your torso, touch your toes). This can kickstart your metabolism and loosen up stiff muscles from sleep.

- **Desk energizer:** Every hour or two at your desk, stand up and move. Do a set of desk stretches – neck rolls, arm circles, reach for the ceiling, gently twist side to side. You can also do chair squats (stand up from your chair and sit back down repeatedly) or desk push-ups (hands on desk, step back and do push-ups). Even 5 minutes of these light exercises will get your blood flowing and help prevent that mid-day slump.

- **Stair climb burst:** If you have stairs in your building, take a quick break to climb briskly for 1-2 minutes. You could simply go up and down one or two flights repeatedly. This will raise your heart rate fast – you might even get a little winded, which is actually the goal for improving cardiovascular fitness in minimal time. Research from the University of Utah found that even a single minute of brisk stair climbing here and there throughout the day was linked to lower odds of weight gain.

- **One-song dance party:** This one's a fan favorite because it's pure fun. Put on an upbeat song – something around 3 to 4 minutes – and dance like crazy. In your living room, in the kitchen while cooking, wherever. Let go and really move: jump, shimmy, twirl, whatever feels good. By the time the song is over, you'll have elevated your heart rate, burned some calories, and likely lifted your mood. It's almost impossible to dance to your favorite tune and *not* feel happier after. Keep a short playlist of go-to "dance break" songs handy for when you need an instant pick-me-up.

- **"Exercise trigger" habit:** Tie a mini-exercise to something you do regularly. For example, every time you hit "Save" on that big project or send a batch of emails, take 2 minutes to do a quick routine: maybe 15 jumping jacks and 15 lunges. Or every time you take a bathroom break, do 10 calf raises while washing your hands. These tiny bits might sound trivial, but remember – they accumulate. Ten calf raises here, 20 jumping jacks there, and by day's end you might have done a couple hundred extra movements.

- **Evening wind-down walk:** After dinner, instead of immediately planting on the couch, take a short walk (even 10 minutes) around the block. This aids digestion, adds to your activity tally, and can segue your mind into relaxation mode for the evening. If weather or darkness is an issue, even walking in place or doing a gentle indoor movement (like light stretching or a mellow yoga flow) for a few minutes helps. Consistency is more important than intensity at night – it's about telling your body that movement is a normal part of your day, morning to night.

Researchers have coined the term "exercise snacking" precisely to emphasize that we can snack on movement throughout the day just as we snack on food. One review found significant benefits on fitness from this approach, including lowered cholesterol and improved cardiovascular function. And a large long-term study observed that people who got just 3-4 minutes of short bursts of activity in daily life (like hurrying to catch a bus or playing with children) had about a 30% reduction in mortality risk related to cardiovascular health, especially among those who weren't doing structured exercise. That's astonishing – *minutes* of effort making a measurable difference in longevity. It reinforces that "60 seconds of vigorous movement still counts". We need to dispel the myth that if you can't do a 30-minute workout, it's not worth doing anything. Science shows *any* movement is better than none, and a little can go a long way when done consistently.

That said, consistency is the secret sauce. Doing an "exercise snack" once in a blue moon won't magically transform your health. The Cleveland Clinic experts note that it's not very impactful if you only do it "when you remember" – the key is making it a daily habit. Try to incorporate a few mini-workouts every day, and aim to keep that up for weeks. You'll likely start noticing you feel fitter and more energetic as the months go by. Many people report that these little bursts also help break up the monotony of work and improve their mood. Dr. Oppezzo from Stanford even suggests that for stress reduction, multiple short bursts might be more effective than one long session: each burst gets your heart rate up and then as you recover, your body enters "calm down" mode, which can reduce overall stress levels when done repeatedly. Essentially, you're training your body to handle spikes of effort and then quickly return to a relaxed state – a sign of good cardiovascular fitness and resilience.

Incorporating "exercise snacks" requires a bit of intention at first, but soon it can become second nature. You might start to actually *crave* these movement breaks because of how refreshed they make you feel. One minute you're lethargic at your desk, then you do a quick set of jumping jacks and voila – you feel more alert than a cup of coffee would make you. It's like pressing a reset button for your body and brain throughout the day.

In summary, no matter how "lazy" or busy you feel, you can embrace the concept of tiny workouts. They are the lazy genius's secret weapon: minimal effort, maximal return. On a super hectic day, maybe all you do is a few five-minute movement breaks – and that is absolutely okay. You're still doing something positive for your health, maintaining the habit of daily activity, and likely boosting your mood and energy to boot. Overachievers often fall into the trap of all-or-nothing, thinking if they can't do a full workout, why bother. But as you now know, *that mindset is outdated.* Even five minutes matters. So embrace the exercise snack. Make movement a series of enjoyable nibbles throughout your day. Your body will thank you, your mind will thank you, and you'll be living proof that fitness truly can fit into *any* life – even one as crazy as yours.

Chapter 5
The Lazy Genius Workout Strategies

In the fitness arena, working smarter beats working longer. This section explores how you can achieve maximum results in minimum time. Gone are the days of believing you must grind for hours at the gym to get fit. Exercise science now shows that brief, efficient workouts can deliver outsized benefits without monopolizing your schedule or breaking your body. By embracing strategies like high-intensity intervals or their gentler alternatives, you'll discover that *you don't need to suffer to get stronger*. Let's dive into the lazy genius approach to exercising effectively, getting fit faster and with far less fuss than you ever thought possible.

Maximum Results, Minimum Time

We live in a busy age, so who wouldn't want a workout that delivers maximum benefits in minimum time? The good news is that fitness researchers have been asking the same question – and the answers are exciting. One of the biggest breakthroughs has been high-intensity interval training (HIIT), which alternates short bursts of *all-out effort* with brief rest periods. HIIT has become wildly popular because it condenses a whole lot of exercise benefit into a small time slot. In fact, according to multiple studies, you can boost your health and fitness "in a matter of minutes" with HIIT. For example, one famous protocol consists of just *20 seconds* of hard work followed by 10 seconds of rest, repeated 8 times

– that's only 4 minutes of exercise – yet it produced greater improvements in aerobic capacity than an hour of traditional moderate cycling. In another study, a "one-minute" interval workout (three 20-second sprints within a 10-minute session, done 3 times a week) improved people's fitness just as much as 50-minute steady workouts done with the same frequency. In short, shortcuts in exercise actually work: a few minutes of pushing yourself can yield the same results as spending five to ten times longer in a typical routine.

Why is HIIT so effective? When you exercise at high intensity (think *sprinting up a hill* or *pedaling a bike as fast as possible*), you challenge your heart, lungs, and muscles in ways that stimulate rapid adaptation. HIIT has been shown to improve cardiovascular health, insulin sensitivity, and cholesterol levels, while also reducing abdominal and visceral fat. It even helps maintain or build muscle mass in less-active individuals – a big plus for anyone looking to get leaner. The magic lies in how HIIT pushes your body: it ramps up your metabolism and can trigger beneficial cellular changes. For instance, intense interval exercise causes your cells' powerhouses (mitochondria) to work more efficiently and even increases their number, which is associated with healthy aging. There's evidence that HIIT may slow down aspects of cellular aging by boosting mitochondrial proteins more effectively than moderate exercise, essentially helping keep your muscles (and possibly other tissues) younger. It's not often you hear a workout being linked to *anti-aging* effects, but these findings underscore just how powerful short, intense exercise can be.

Of course, if HIIT sounds too good to be true, there is a small catch: it's hard work. Those few minutes of all-out effort *will* feel challenging – after all, you're asking your body to push near its limits. In practice, 30 seconds of an all-out sprint can feel like forever when your lungs and legs are burning. Not everyone enjoys that level of intensity, and it's perfectly okay if you don't. Exercise should not be a *"grueling survival test"* every time. In fact, experts emphasize that *"exercise DOESN'T have to be a grueling"* ordeal to be effective. If you try HIIT and find it leaves you feeling faint or overly stressed, you're not alone – researchers have noted that some participants feel dizzy or even occasionally *get ill* when first adapting to super-intense workouts. Moreover, doing HIIT too often can increase injury risk or simply burn you out. Your body needs recovery time after such taxing efforts, which is why trainers typically recommend not doing HIIT every day (often no more than 2-3 times per week with rest in between). So, while HIIT can quickly whip you into shape, it's not mandatory for everyone, especially if you dread it or it doesn't suit your current fitness level.

Enter the concept of LIIT – Low-Intensity Interval Training, HIIT's gentler cousin. LIIT follows a similar idea of interval-based exercise but dials down the intensity so that it's much more comfortable and sustainable. Instead of sprinting breathlessly, a LIIT workout might have you exercise at a *moderate pace* for a few minutes, then take a short rest, and repeat. You're still alternating effort and recovery, but at an intensity where you can hold a conversation and your heart rate stays in a moderate zone. The result? You still get fitter, but without the gasping and pain. Fitness experts describe LIIT as "challenging yourself a little bit" with an effort level you can sustain longer. Because you're not maxing out, LIIT sessions tend to last longer than HIIT – perhaps 20, 30, or even 40 minutes – but they feel much easier on the body. This means *far less wear and tear*: with LIIT, you won't be excessively sore the next day and you likely won't need as many days off to recover. In fact, minimal recovery time is a key benefit – you're able to exercise again sooner because you haven't traumatized your muscles. LIIT significantly reduces injury risk as well, since you avoid the extreme forces and exhaustion that can cause form to break down. For anyone who's been injured or is wary of high-impact training, LIIT offers a *lower-risk path* to fitness.

Now, you might wonder: can easier workouts really give results comparable to HIIT? Research suggests that yes, you can achieve similar improvements, as long as you adjust the duration. Think of intensity and time as a trade-off: if you go *harder*, you can afford to go shorter; if you go *easier*, you should go a bit longer. For example, one analysis noted that if a typical HIIT session is 15 minutes, a LIIT session might need to be around 30 minutes to burn a similar amount of calories. Over the long run, studies have found that low-intensity exercise can reduce body fat about as much as high-intensity exercise, provided the energy expenditure is equivalent. The higher intensities do tend to boost aerobic fitness and certain health markers a bit more quickly, but both approaches are beneficial. Most importantly, *LIIT proves that you don't have to punish yourself to get stronger and healthier.* "No pain, no gain" is outdated thinking – exercise can (and maybe should) feel good while still delivering gains. One exercise physiologist put it plainly: *"Turning down the intensity on exercise doesn't turn off the advantages."* You still get improvements in heart health, weight management, mood and more by doing regular moderate workouts. In fact, doing workouts you enjoy (or at least can tolerate) means you'll stick with them longer, which is the real secret to seeing results.

The lazy genius takeaway here is one of efficiency and personalization. If you're an overachiever short on time, HIIT offers a proven shortcut to better fitness – you can literally squeeze a day's worth of cardio into a coffee break. On the other hand, if you're a bit of a burnout or someone who *hates the gym torture*, LIIT is your friend – you can get fit with *less strain and stress*, perhaps by taking brisk walk-jog intervals in the park or doing a low-impact circuit while watching TV. Either way, you're maximizing the benefit for the time you invest. Remember, the goal isn't to brag about how long you spent working out or how brutally hard it was; the goal is to *feel healthier, get stronger, and stay sane*. Science is unequivocal: you can absolutely achieve those goals without spending hours in the gym. By leveraging interval techniques – whether intense or gentle – you'll prove to yourself that sometimes *less really is more*.

Strength Training Made Simple

For many busy people, the idea of strength training conjures images of bodybuilders pumping iron for hours or complicated gym machines that target dozens of muscle groups. It's no surprise that overachievers short on time often feel strength workouts are too time-consuming or complex to squeeze in. But here's the reality: building strength doesn't have to be a big production. A lazy genius knows how to get strong with minimal fuss. In this section, we demystify strength training and offer simple strategies to build muscle and boost your metabolism without living at the gym. The truth is that you can gain strength and lean muscle in just a couple of brief sessions per week – no grueling six-day bodybuilding schedule required! By focusing on a few key principles and "hacks," even the busiest person can incorporate strength training into their wellness plan and reap huge benefits.

First, let's talk about why you'd bother with strength training at all. If your goal is to get healthy and "fit" overall, resistance exercise is a crucial piece of the puzzle. Aerobic exercise (like running or cycling) gets most of the spotlight for heart health, but strength training provides unique benefits that cardio alone can't. When you challenge your muscles – whether with weights, resistance bands, or just your body weight – you help preserve and build lean muscle mass, which naturally declines with age. More muscle doesn't just make you stronger; it also raises your metabolic rate, meaning you burn more calories even at rest. This can be a game-changer for weight management: by doing a bit of strength work, you essentially turn your body into a more efficient calorie-burning machine throughout the day. Strength training also strengthens your bones (warding off osteoporosis), protects your joints, and improves balance and functional ability. Research has even linked regular strength exercise to lower risks of heart disease, diabetes, and other chronic conditions. Perhaps most impressively, building some muscle could literally help you live longer. A large analysis found that people who did just *30–60 minutes of muscle-strengthening activities per week* had significantly lower risk of premature death, including from cancer and heart disease.

The benefits plateaued after about an hour per week, which means you don't need endless training – *around two sessions per week was enough to make a big difference*. In fact, authorities like the U.S. Department of Health and Human Services recommend strength training all major muscle groups at least two times a week as part of a balanced exercise routine. The bottom line is clear: a little strength training goes a long way for your health.

So how can we make strength training *simple and time-efficient?* One lazy-genius approach is to focus on compound movements. Compound exercises are those that engage multiple muscle groups in one move. Think of exercises like squats, push-ups, lunges, pull-ups, or rows. When you do a squat, for example, you're not only working your quadriceps (front thighs), but also glutes, hamstrings, core, and even your back to stabilize. With a single exercise, you hit a whole network of muscles. This is much more efficient than isolation exercises (like a bicep curl that only works one small area). A few compound movements can give you a *full-body workout* in a short time. For instance, a 20-minute session at home could include push-ups (for chest, shoulders, and triceps), bodyweight squats or chair squats (for legs and glutes), bent-over rows with dumbbells or resistance bands (for back and biceps), and planks (for core). In just four exercises you've engaged nearly every major muscle. This kind of routine is perfect for an overachiever who wants the biggest payoff for their time invested.

Another key strategy is to take advantage of bodyweight exercises and simple equipment. You don't need an expensive gym or fancy machines to build strength. Your own body provides plenty of resistance. Classic moves like push-ups, pull-ups, planks, and tricep dips can be done anywhere and can be modified to suit your level (e.g. doing push-ups on your knees or against a wall if you're just starting). Resistance bands are another "lazy" tool – they are cheap, portable, and effective for adding extra challenge to movements like rows, presses, or leg exercises. Even improvised weights can work: for example, using a pair of heavy books or water bottles as dumbbells for some curls or shoulder presses. The goal is to remove barriers and keep it simple. If you can roll out of bed and do a quick bodyweight circuit in your living room, you're more likely to actually do it, versus a complicated plan that requires driving to the gym and remembering a dozen machine settings. The lazy genius embraces the motto: *the simplest plan is the one you'll stick with.* And consistency beats perfection.

Speaking of simplicity, here's a liberating fact backed by science: you don't have to do endless sets and reps to get results. Many people assume you must do multiple sets of an exercise (say 3 sets of 10 reps each) to build muscle. While that's a traditional approach, research shows that a single set of an exercise, performed with proper intensity, can be *just as effective* as multiple sets for strength gains. The key is to work that set to muscle fatigue – meaning you choose a resistance that makes the last rep difficult to complete with good form. If you hit that point, your muscle has received a strong stimulus to adapt and grow, whether you did one set or three. For most people aiming for general fitness, one focused set per exercise is sufficient. This is fantastic news for the time-crunched: it literally cuts your workout time by two-thirds without sacrificing results. For example, instead of doing 3 sets of 15 bodyweight squats spread out with rest, you could do one set of 20–25 squats *until your legs really feel it*, and then move on. You'll still reap strength gains, and you've saved time. Similarly, experts note you can see significant improvements in strength with just two or three 20–30 minute strength sessions per week. You read that right – *less than an hour per week of strength training can do the job.* There's even evidence (especially in beginners or older adults) that training once a week can increase strength nearly as much as training twice or three times weekly. Knowing this, you can banish the guilt that you're "supposed" to be in the weight room every day. Instead, schedule a couple of short sessions for strength and feel great about it – it's truly all you need for robust benefits.

To make those brief sessions count, here are a few lazy genius tips:

- **Prioritize form and quality over quantity.** Move slowly and with control, really feeling the target muscles work. A well-executed set of 10 quality push-ups is better than flailing through 20 half-reps.

- **Use the heaviest resistance that allows you to complete your reps with good form.** This might mean using a heavier dumbbell for fewer reps, or just doing bodyweight but very slow tempo. The idea is to reach that challenging fatigue point by the end of your set. If you breeze through 15 reps with energy to spare, it's time to increase the difficulty (add weight, or do a harder variation).

- **Incorporate full-body moves** when possible (e.g. a squat with an overhead press combines lower and upper body in one move). This raises the intensity and efficiency.

- **Give yourself rest days** for the muscles you worked. Muscles actually get stronger during recovery, so take at least a day off before working the same muscle group again. With only two or three sessions a week, this is easy to manage. On off-days, you can focus on cardio or mobility, or simply rest.

Finally, remember that the goal of strength training for wellness isn't to become the next Mr. or Ms. Olympia; it's to enhance your life. With minimal time investment, you'll start to notice daily tasks feeling easier – carrying groceries, climbing stairs, even sitting with good posture. You'll likely see changes in your physique too: muscles slightly more defined, posture more confident. And the metabolic boost will help in managing weight over time. All of that can be achieved with a no-frills routine that fits into your week with ease. The lazy genius knows that simplicity and consistency beat complicated routines that you can't maintain. So go ahead and embrace strength training made simple – your future self (with stronger bones, toned muscles, and a faster metabolism) will thank you for it, and you'll barely have had to break a sweat in terms of time spent.

Smart Tech and Tools (In Moderation)

Technology has transformed nearly every aspect of our lives, and fitness is no exception. For the lazy genius looking to stay motivated, smart tech and tools can be a game-changer – when used wisely. This section explores how gadgets and apps can inject fun, accountability, and personalization into your workouts, essentially gamifying exercise so it doesn't feel like a chore. But we'll also discuss the flip side: too much tech can lead to information overload or anxiety. The goal is to leverage technology as a helpful servant, not let it become a tyrannical master that dictates your every move. When used in moderation, fitness tech can support your journey and even make you *enjoy* staying active.

One of the most accessible tools is the smartphone in your pocket. There's a plethora of fitness apps that can guide you through workouts, track your progress, and reward you with virtual badges. For example, apps can put together quick HIIT routines or yoga sessions on demand, so you don't have to figure out what to do – you just follow along. Many overachievers love the sense of structure and data these apps provide: you can see how many workouts you've done this month, how your running pace improves, or how much weight you've lifted over time. Wearable fitness trackers take it a step further by tracking your activity continuously. Devices like Fitbit, Apple Watch, or Garmin watches count your steps, monitor heart rate, estimate calories burned, and even remind you to stand up if you've been sitting too long. This kind of feedback can be incredibly motivating. Studies indicate that these devices *often do nudge people toward healthier habits*, at least initially. For someone with a desk job, a gentle buzz on the wrist to "move for a few minutes" each hour can help break up sedentary time. Over the course of a day, those little bits of movement add up. Many trackers also let you join challenges with friends – who can get the most steps this week? – which turns fitness into a friendly competition.

Speaking of competition and fun, a rising trend is exergaming – using video games that require physical activity. If you're someone who hates traditional exercise, you might find that *playing a game* distracts you from the fact you're actually working out. There are many examples of this: dancing games that score your moves, virtual reality boxing or sword-fighting games that have you ducking, squatting and punching, or even mobile phone games like augmented reality scavenger hunts that make you walk around your city. Active video games can be surprisingly effective workouts. One study cited by experts showed that certain active games can improve strength and cardiorespiratory fitness in older adults, not just kids. They're also associated with more positive mood during exercise, which is important because enjoying your workout means you'll stick with it longer. Gamifying your exercise taps into the human love of play and reward. As one sports medicine physician put it, *"Exergaming embodies the idea that staying healthy should be accessible, achievable and — most importantly — enjoyable for everyone."* In other words, working out doesn't have to feel like work – it can feel like leveling up in a game. For instance, a game like Ring Fit Adventure turns strength and cardio exercises into an adventure quest; you defeat enemies by performing squats or overhead presses. Other games give you points or trophies for hitting certain targets. These elements give a sense of accomplishment beyond just calories or time – you're focusing on beating the game, and *"calories are burned — all without feeling like a workout"*. Exergaming can also be very approachable for beginners; if you're intimidated by the gym, stepping into a virtual world where you're slaying dragons with lunges can be a much gentler entry point. Importantly, the fun factor can make you forget you're exercising, reducing stress and even improving mental health while you move.

Fitness technology can make workouts feel like play: for example, virtual reality and active video games turn exercise into an immersive, fun experience that keeps you moving without "forcing" it. Beyond games, even simple tech tools like music playlists can enhance your workouts. Creating a high-energy playlist that times with your interval runs or a calming playlist for stretching can boost your performance and enjoyment. There are also smart home gym systems now – mirrors or apps that give real-time feedback on your form, or stationary bikes that simulate racing others in a virtual landscape. All these innovations can be great motivational tricks. They keep you engaged, provide structure, and satisfy that inner data-geek by showing progress in numbers and charts.

However, here's where the caution comes in: tech should empower you, not overwhelm you. It's easy to fall into the trap of obsessing over numbers – whether it's steps, calories, heart rate zones, or sleep scores. Many of us have felt that twinge of guilt when our smartwatch shows we didn't hit 10,000 steps today. But consider this: the famous "10,000 steps" goal didn't even come from medical science – it started as a marketing slogan for a pedometer in 1964! In reality, studies have found that significantly fewer steps (e.g. around 7,000 per day) can still dramatically lower mortality risk. Yet the allure of that round number can make us feel like failures on days we fall short. The lazy genius perspective is to *use* the data without letting it judge you. Don't become a slave to arbitrary goals. If a tracker motivates you to walk more, fantastic – but if you find yourself, say, marching around your bedroom at midnight just to see "100% of goal" on your app, it might be time to loosen the tech's grip on your life.

Experts have noted that while tracking metrics can motivate, it can also lead to unhealthy fixation or anxiety in some people. There's even a term "data overload": modern devices spew out so much information – heart rate, sleep quality, VO2 max, stress level – that you can feel overwhelmed trying to make sense of it all. If you start believing you must optimize every metric, the process of getting healthy ironically can make you *mentally* less healthy by generating constant worry. For instance, one journal study found that patients using wearables to monitor a heart condition ended up more anxious because every little fluctuation in data made them fret something was wrong. Therapists have seen cases where people become obsessed with burning a certain number of calories or feel panic if their watch's rings aren't all closed by end of day. This is the opposite of what we want – fitness tech should be serving your wellness, not undermining it.

So how do we keep tech as a *servant*? The key is moderation and mindful use. Here are a few tips:

- **Choose the metrics that matter to you**, and ignore the rest. Maybe you care about getting 30 minutes of activity a day, but you don't need to monitor your exact heart rate variability. Tailor your app settings and dashboard to show what motivates you and hide what confuses or stresses you.

- **Set boundaries on when you check your data.** Constantly glancing at your step count or calorie burn can create a neurotic feedback loop. Perhaps look at your stats *once a day* or review the week as a whole, rather than reacting in real-time to every dip and peak.

- **Use tech for positive reinforcement, not punishment.** Celebrate the milestones and streaks (e.g. when your app congratulates you for exercising 5 days this week). But if you miss a goal, practice self-compassion. Remember that these goals are somewhat arbitrary – what matters is the trend of staying active over time, not a single day's numbers.

- **Take tech breaks** when needed. If you feel yourself becoming too dependent, try working out without your devices occasionally. Go for a run with no watch and just tune into your body's signals – how you feel is more important than the exact pace. One therapist advises creating *"tech-free zones"* or times, so you can reconnect with the joy of movement unmediated by gadgets.

- **Keep perspective: data is just data**. As one expert said, *"We don't want to be so data-driven that we forget to be human."* Your fitness journey is a human experience, not a spreadsheet. The numbers are tools, but they never tell the whole story of your effort, improvements, or how exercise makes you feel.

In summary, smart tech and fitness tools can greatly enhance your motivation and enjoyment – they can turn a solo workout into a social game, provide guidance like a personal trainer in your pocket, and reinforce your good habits with gratifying stats. Embrace these benefits, especially if you're someone who loves gamification or needs that extra push. But also give yourself permission to *step back* from the metrics if they start to steal the joy or add stress. Use tech on your own terms: let it *remind* you to be active, let it *celebrate* your progress, but never let it guilt or boss you around. By striking this balance, you'll have the best of both worlds – high-tech support with low-stress attitude – truly a lazy genius way to stay fit.

Habit Stacking for Fitness

One of the biggest challenges for busy people is finding time for regular workouts. You've got work, family, and countless responsibilities vying for your attention. Too often, exercise becomes an afterthought – something you *intend* to do if time permits (and let's be honest, time usually doesn't permit). The lazy genius solution? Stop treating workouts as an optional add-on and instead build them into your routine through "habit stacking." This approach involves attaching a small exercise habit onto something you already do every day, so that being active becomes as automatic as brushing your teeth or having your morning coffee. In this section, we'll present practical tips to fit workouts into a packed schedule by piggybacking on your existing habits. By doing this, you cement consistency almost effortlessly, turning fitness from a daunting task into an integrated part of your day.

So what exactly is habit stacking? It's a term popularized by author James Clear in *Atomic Habits*, but the concept is simple and has been around in psychology for a long time. Habit stacking means pairing a new desired behavior with an existing habit or cue. You're effectively saying: *"After/Before I do [everyday habit], I will do [new habit]."* The reason this works is that your current habits are already wired into your brain; you do them consistently without much thought (think about how automatically you put on a seatbelt when you get in a car, or boil water for tea in the morning). By latching a new action onto that solid anchor, you're more likely to remember and actually do it. The existing habit serves as a trigger. Over time, the new habit gets reinforced and becomes part of that routine sequence. It's like sneaking a new ingredient into a recipe you cook daily – eventually it becomes a standard part of the recipe.

When it comes to fitness, habit stacking can be a game-changer for consistency. Instead of trying to carve out a big chunk of time for the gym (which often gets postponed or cancelled due to a busy schedule), you insert *mini-workouts into moments that already exist.* Think in terms of tiny exercises attached to daily rituals. For example:

- **Morning coffee brew + movement**: While waiting for your coffee to brew or tea to steep, do a set of lunges or squats. It might be 1-2 minutes of exercise, but done daily it adds up.

- **Brushing your teeth + exercise**: As you brush your teeth (a solid two minutes, we hope), you can do a wall sit – back against the wall, knees bent – holding that position until you're done brushing. Or do calf raises or single-leg balances. You're literally strengthening your legs while cleaning your teeth.

- **Walking the dog + extra steps**: If you let the dog out in the yard each morning, do a quick burst of jumping jacks or jog in place while Fido sniffs around. The dog might give you a funny look, but your heart will thank you.

- **Phone calls + stretching**: Every time you have a work call (if it's audio only), use a headset and pace or do simple stretches during the conversation. You've stacked movement onto a routine task.

- **TV time + floor exercises**: Make it a habit that whenever you watch your favorite show in the evening, you'll do something like planks or yoga stretches during the first commercial break (or every 15 minutes if streaming without ads).

- **Stairs habit**: Attach a habit that whenever you need to go upstairs at home, you always take two trips – one extra up-and-down for bonus exercise. Climbing stairs is terrific cardio and leg work packed into a short burst.

By implementing these kinds of tiny combos, you integrate fitness into your life stealthily. You hardly notice the effort because it's woven into something you're already doing. As one guide put it, *"habit stacking camouflages the new-to-you task into your normal, everyday behaviors"*, making the healthy action "just a simple part of a daily to-do you're already comfortable with." In other words, the new exercise habit rides on the coattails of an established routine, which makes it *feel less intrusive*.

The beauty of habit stacking is that it works for multiple small habits once you get the hang of it. Maybe you start with one (say, push-ups after your morning coffee). Once that becomes second nature, you can stack another, like doing a quick yoga stretch sequence right after you shut down your computer at work each day. Over time, you create a *"tower" of healthy habits* linked to your daily anchors. But be cautious not to stack too much at once; build gradually so you don't overwhelm yourself.

While the small daily moves are fantastic, what about stacking for more substantial workouts? You can also use the principle to ensure you get your dedicated workout sessions done by tying them to a regular event. For instance, if you notice you often have some free time or a dip in emails after lunch, make it a habit that right after lunch on Mondays, Wednesdays, and Fridays, you go for a 20-minute walk or do a short gym session. The after-lunch routine becomes your cue – just like brushing teeth is a cue – that signals "time to move." If you're a morning person, you could stack "after I drop the kids at school, I will do a 15-minute workout video." If you have more energy in the evening, maybe "immediately when I get home from work, I change into workout clothes and do a quick weights session *before* I relax or start dinner." The exact scheduling will depend on your personal rhythms, but the idea is to schedule workouts when you naturally have the most energy and likelihood to follow through. Research and common experience suggest that many people find morning works best, since fewer distractions have popped up yet and it sets a positive tone for the day. Morning exercisers also tend to be more consistent, partly because nothing (meetings, fatigue, social invites) has had a chance to derail the plan. But if you are *not* a morning person, don't force it. You might stack exercise onto your lunch break or early evening when you feel most alert. The consensus among experts is that *"the best time to exercise is when you have the most energy and motivation to do it"* – for some that's sunrise, for others it's after work. Choose the time you can stick with, and then make it a ritual, just like you wouldn't skip brushing your teeth. By doing so, you remove the mental debate each day ("should I work out now or later?") and instead it's just *part of what you do*, almost as automatic as habit as any other daily task.

To successfully habit-stack your way into fitness, keep these tips in mind:

- **Start small and specific.** If you try to stack a 30-minute workout onto a habit, it might not stick initially because it's a big ask. Instead, start with something that takes 1-5 minutes. For example, "after I take my morning shower, I'll do 10 push-ups" is concrete and small. You can always expand it later.

- **Use immediate triggers.** The new habit should follow the existing one *immediately* or at least be clearly connected. "After I pour my coffee, I will do squats" works because it's immediate. "After breakfast sometime before work, I'll exercise" is too vague – your brain won't hook into it.

- **Track and celebrate** your streaks initially. Put a little checkmark on a calendar for each day you succeed in stacking your mini-workout. This creates a satisfying visual chain and you'll be motivated not to break it. Even though it's "lazy" in concept, you'll feel proud of these small wins.

- **Adjust if needed.** If one stack isn't working (maybe you're too groggy to do push-ups *right* after waking up), don't give up on stacking – just try a different pairing or time. Perhaps you find you're more willing after your first cup of coffee. Find what flows naturally.

Over time, these mini-habits can ignite bigger changes. You might find that 10 push-ups after coffee becomes easy, so you bump it to 15, then 20, or you add a second exercise. Or maybe consistently walking 10 minutes after dinner evolves into a routine where some evenings you feel like extending it to 30 minutes because you're enjoying it. Small steps have a way of snowballing into significant progress when done consistently. This is the essence of the lazy genius philosophy: by embedding fitness into your daily life in modest ways, you remove the hardest part – which is *getting started*. There's no mental battle to go to the gym; you're already in motion as part of something you do, and before you know it, exercise is just another habit – as routine as checking your email.

In conclusion, habit stacking allows even the busiest, most "over it" individuals to make fitness a seamless part of life. Instead of hoping for large blocks of free time (which may never come), you capitalize on the habits and schedule you already have. The result is consistency – those little daily doses of movement keep you active and gradually improve your strength, flexibility, and endurance. Perhaps most importantly, this approach reinforces the identity of an active person. You'll start to see yourself as someone who *moves regularly*, almost unconsciously, rather than someone who "can't find time to exercise." And that identity shift is powerful. It means fitness is no longer something on your to-do list – *it's woven into the fabric of your day*. With habit stacking, you truly embody the idea of "The Anti-Hustle Health Plan": you're not hustling to get to a gym or punish yourself in massive workouts. You're sneaking health and fitness into your life cleverly and effortlessly, allowing you to get fit, stay sane, and actually enjoy your life – all at the same time.

Chapter 6

Eat to Nourish and Enjoy

Throwing Out the Diet Rulebook

Toxic diet culture convinces us that wellness means rigid rules and "all or nothing" eating, but this approach often backfires. When you follow an extremely restrictive diet – cutting out entire food groups or severely slashing calories – it may work for a short time, but the rebound can be brutal. Studies show that most dieters regain the weight they lose, and many end up heavier than when they started. In fact, strict diets trigger psychological effects like intense cravings for the "forbidden" foods, constant preoccupation with eating, and eventual bingeing once willpower snaps. In other words, the very strategy meant to control your eating can lead to feeling out of control. Dieting isn't just joyless – it's ineffective in the long run, with research indicating that it usually fails to produce lasting weight loss and can even predict future weight gain.

One reason traditional diets fail is the "what-the-hell effect," a phenomenon where one slip-up leads to a spiral of overeating. Psychologists have observed that if people on a diet believe they've broken a rule (say, by eating a slice of pizza), they often throw in the towel and eat far more afterward than they otherwise would. This all-or-nothing thinking – viewing yourself as either *perfectly compliant* or a *failure*

– undermines healthy intentions. It creates a cycle of guilt and overindulgence: you skip the office cake for weeks, but when you finally give in one day, you figure "I've blown it, so I might as well go all out." Such cycles erode self-trust and make eating feel like a battleground rather than a normal part of life. Moreover, chronic restrictive dieting is linked with higher stress hormones and even symptoms of depression as your body and mind rebel against constant deprivation. Clearly, fighting yourself with ever-stricter food rules is a losing game for both your health and happiness.

It's time to reject that punitive diet mentality and embrace a more sustainable, kind approach to eating. Enter intuitive eating – a science-backed alternative that throws out the rigid rulebook and teaches you to tune into your body's natural signals. Intuitive eating means eating when you're hungry, choosing foods that satisfy you, and stopping when you're comfortably full, rather than when an external diet plan tells you to. This approach actively encourages rejecting the notion of "good" and "bad" foods. By listening to internal hunger and fullness cues instead of following strict menus or calorie counts, people learn to trust themselves around food again. Far from being a free-for-all, intuitive eating is about relearning what *healthy* feels like for *your* body. Remarkably, research shows that intuitive eaters tend to have better psychological health and a lower likelihood of disordered eating behaviors compared to chronic dieters. In one long-term study, adolescents who scored higher on intuitive eating had significantly lower odds of developing binge-eating habits or extreme weight control behaviors by young adulthood. They also reported fewer depressive symptoms and higher self-esteem, highlighting how closely our relationship with food ties into mental well-being. The takeaway is powerful: you can eat well without militant rules. By honoring your body's needs – eating when hungry, choosing nourishing foods that you truly enjoy, and stopping when satisfied – you'll nourish yourself in a way that is physically sustainable and emotionally sane. Ditching diet-culture extremes for an intuitive, balanced mindset is not about giving up; it's about gaining freedom. You learn that you haven't "failed" if you eat a cookie; you've simply eaten something tasty, and you can trust your body to guide the next meal. In rejecting the all-or-nothing mentality, you'll find a healthier middle ground where good nutrition and enjoyment happily co-exist.

Simplified Nutrition for Busy Lives

Healthy eating often gets cast as a time-consuming chore – endless meal prep, complicated recipes, expensive shopping lists. But nourishing yourself does not require perfection or hours in the kitchen each day. In fact, a few *lazy-genius* hacks can streamline nutrition for even the busiest schedule, yielding big benefits in your energy and health with minimal hassle. The secret is to be strategic and kind to yourself: make simple changes that fit into your life, rather than trying to force an unrealistic meal-plan overhaul. With a handful of smart shortcuts, you can fuel your body well even when you're short on time (or motivation).

To start, embrace the power of efficiency in meal planning – think "cook once, eat twice." If you're cooking anyway, why not make a double batch? Prepare a large casserole or a whole roasting tray of veggies and protein when you have time, and enjoy the leftovers the next day so you get two homemade meals for the effort of one. For example, grill or bake extra chicken breasts on Sunday and toss the extra into a salad or wrap on Monday. A big pot of chili or stir-fry can be lunch for tomorrow. By intentionally cooking in bulk, you avoid having to reinvent the wheel (or heat up the stove) every single day. Along with batch cooking, stock your kitchen with time-saving ingredients. Frozen or pre-cut vegetables are a busy cook's best friend – they provide the same nutrients as fresh produce, but save you the washing and chopping. You can throw a handful of frozen broccoli or a pre-chopped stir-fry mix into a pan and have a dinner ready in minutes. Similarly, keep staples like canned beans on hand; they're packed with protein and fiber, cost less than meat, and require no soaking or boiling – just rinse and add to your dish. These convenient options eliminate the usual prep work, so a healthy meal is never far away, even when you're exhausted after work.

In fact, fueling yourself well can be as simple as assembling a few basic building blocks. You don't need elaborate recipes every night – rely on a rotation of quick, healthy meals that you enjoy and know how to make. Maybe it's a vegetable omelet, a hearty salad with lots of toppings, a stir-fry with frozen veggies, or a one-pot soup. Pick a few go-to options and repeat them often. This kind of meal rotation reduces decision fatigue (no more agonizing over "What's for dinner?" each evening) and ensures you always have the ingredients you need. And remember, shortcuts are absolutely allowed. Use that rotisserie chicken from the grocery store as the protein for tonight's grain bowl. Toss pre-washed greens in a bowl with cherry tomatoes and canned chickpeas for a five-minute salad. There is zero shame in using prepared items to save time –

it's a smart way to make healthy eating fit into a busy life. By removing the pressure to cook everything from scratch, you make it much more likely that you'll stick to nourishing choices instead of resorting to fast food or skipping meals.

Here are some lazy-genius nutrition hacks to streamline healthy eating on a tight schedule:

- **Plan for leftovers:** Whenever you cook, make extra. A big batch of food (like a stew, grain dish, or roast veggies) can be packed for tomorrow's lunch or reinvented for dinner on another night. This "cook once, eat twice" strategy saves time and ensures you always have something nutritious on hand.

- **Stock shortcut ingredients:** Keep a supply of quick-to-use foods in your kitchen. For example, buy pre-washed salad greens and frozen mixed vegetables for instant vitamins, and keep canned beans or tuna for easy protein. With these staples, you can throw together a balanced meal with almost no prep – think a veggie-packed omelet or a burrito bowl – faster than waiting for takeout.

- **Rotate simple recipes:** Develop a small repertoire of easy, healthy recipes that you enjoy and can make on autopilot. It could be as simple as whole-grain pasta with sautéed veggies, a quinoa salad with chopped nuts and dried fruit, or a quick stir-fry with tofu. Having 5–7 trusty meals in rotation removes the stress on busy nights because you know exactly how to whip them up.

- **Use smart grocery shortcuts:** Let the store do some of the work for you. It's perfectly fine to use pre-cut fruits and veggies, bottled minced garlic, or a healthy frozen entrée in a pinch. You can augment convenience items with fresh components – for instance, add a bag of pre-cut stir-fry veggies to a ready-made teriyaki sauce and protein. By combining convenience foods with whole ingredients, you get a meal that's both fast and nourishing, no perfection required.

By implementing even a couple of these strategies, you'll notice that eating well starts feeling *easier*. The key is consistency, not complexity. Maybe you begin by prepping lunch for two days of the week, or swapping your usual drive-thru breakfast for a quick banana and peanut butter toast at home. Such changes might seem small, but they add up. In fact, nutrition experts emphasize that small, sustainable changes can lead to big benefits in your health and energy over time. You don't need an "all-or-nothing" overhaul – gradual improvements not only boost your well-being, they're also more likely to stick. Perhaps you'll find that having balanced meals ready actually *gives* you more energy to tackle your busy day, creating a positive cycle. By simplifying nutrition to fit your life, you prove that a hectic schedule is not a barrier to wellness. With efficient planning and a forgiving mindset, you can keep yourself well-fueled and feeling your best, no matter how full your calendar is.

Food and Mood

Eating isn't just about fueling your body or managing your weight – it has a profound impact on how you feel day to day. Food is essentially a source of information for your brain and nervous system. The nutrients (or lack thereof) in your meals can influence your energy levels, mental focus, and even your emotional outlook. Have you ever noticed how an afternoon of sugary snacks can leave you irritable and foggy, while a balanced lunch makes you feel steady and clear-headed? This is the food-mood connection in action. In fact, large-scale research has started to confirm what many of us sense intuitively: a balanced diet is linked to better mental health and sharper cognitive function. In one 2024 study of over 180,000 people, those who followed a well-rounded eating pattern (with a mix of vegetables, fruits, proteins, and whole grains) tended to have lower rates of depression and anxiety and performed better on tests of focus and memory. Nutrition, it turns out, isn't just about keeping your body fit – it's also about keeping your mind bright and happy.

One important way food affects mood and mental energy is through blood sugar stability. When we consume refined carbs or sugary foods alone (think candy, white bread, soda), they digest quickly and cause blood sugar to spike. You might feel a brief burst of energy, but what goes up must come down – a rapid insulin response drives that sugar out of the blood, and your levels can drop sharply within a short time. The result? A classic sugar crash, leaving you shaky, drained, and unable to concentrate about 30 minutes after the sweet treat. These sudden highs and lows in blood glucose can make mood and energy levels yo-yo dramatically through the day. To avoid the rollercoaster, focus on steady fuel: pair carbohydrates with protein and fiber, and opt for complex carbs that digest more slowly. For example, instead of a pastry by itself in the mid-morning, have a piece of whole-grain toast with almond butter, or some yogurt with fruit. The protein and healthy fat help slow digestion, leading to a more gradual release of glucose into your bloodstream. This means more sustained energy and no sudden crash. Nutrition experts note that combining fiber-rich carbs with lean proteins and good fats at meals is a winning formula – it prevents blood sugar spikes and keeps you feeling full and focused for longer. A balanced breakfast of oats with nuts and berries, or eggs with whole-grain toast and avocado, will carry you calmly through the morning hours, whereas a sugary cereal might have you ravenous and cranky by 10 a.m. By planning meals and snacks with an eye toward blood sugar balance, you'll likely notice more consistent energy and a brighter mood throughout your day.

Another tip for maintaining stable energy is don't skip meals, especially if you're busy. It's easy to get caught up in work and push through lunch, but running on empty can set you up for mood swings and brain fog. Skipping any meal – particularly breakfast – has been shown to impair your ability to focus and solve problems because your brain isn't getting the steady supply of nutrients it needs. Many people who routinely skip meals end up overeating later or grabbing quick high-sugar snacks, which only exacerbates the energy swings. You can prevent that afternoon slump and the 3 p.m. crankiness by eating regular, balanced meals. Include some protein (to keep hunger at bay) and complex carbs (for fuel) in each meal. For instance, adding chicken or tofu to your salad at lunch and including a piece of fruit or some brown rice will give you both immediate and sustained energy. Also be mindful of caffeine and hydration – while a cup of coffee can boost alertness, overdoing caffeine and forgetting water can leave you jittery or sluggish. Often a mid-afternoon bout of fatigue is partly dehydration, so drinking water steadily during the day is key for concentration and mood as well. In short, nourishing your body at regular intervals and with the right balance sets the stage for mental clarity and emotional steadiness, which is just as important as any number on the scale.

Notably, the food-mood connection extends beyond energy swings to longer-term mental well-being. A growing field of "nutritional psychiatry" explores how diet quality correlates with risks of depression and anxiety. The findings are encouraging: diets rich in whole foods – vegetables, fruits, whole grains, lean proteins, and healthy fats – are associated with lower rates of mood disorders, whereas diets high in ultra-processed foods, sugars, and unhealthy fats are linked to higher rates of these issues. For example, researchers have found that people who eat plenty of fruits and leafy greens tend to report less anxiety, and one reason is the steady supply of vitamins and antioxidants that support brain health. On the flip side, a diet full of fried foods and sugary treats might increase inflammation and oxidative stress in the body, which some studies suggest can negatively affect the brain and mood regulation. There's also the aspect of nutrient deficiencies – lacking certain nutrients like B vitamins, iron, or omega-3 fatty acids can leave you feeling tired and blue. A balanced diet helps cover those bases, contributing to a more stable and positive mood. Additionally, complex carbohydrates (like those in whole grains and legumes) actually help the brain produce serotonin, a neurotransmitter that promotes calm and happiness. That's one reason why a bowl of whole-grain pasta or oatmeal can have a soothing effect: complex carbs are metabolized slowly and keep blood sugar even, which creates a calmer physiological state. Eating this way, especially combined with not going too long without food, may reduce jitteriness and stress signals in the body. Of course, food is not a magic cure for serious anxiety or depression, but it's empowering to know that nourishing yourself can be one tool in your toolkit for better mental health. You're not just *feeding* your body – you're also tending to your mind and mood with each balanced meal.

Ultimately, paying attention to nutrition is about feeling your best. When you supply your body with wholesome foods in a regular, balanced way, you're likely to notice you have more stable energy (no more nodding off in meetings), improved concentration, and even better sleep at night. Many people report that when they clean up their eating habits, they feel less anxious and more emotionally even-keeled, as if a low-level fog has lifted. Science backs up these anecdotes: for instance, one large study noted that individuals on a balanced diet not only had fewer mental health struggles, but they performed better on cognitive tasks – essentially, they could think faster and remember more, a testament to the power of good fuel. So as you design your anti-hustle health plan, remember that nutrition isn't just about nutrients; it's about quality of life. By eating in a way that nourishes and stabilizes you, you're investing in a calmer mind and a more resilient mood. The bottom line: food is mood. Every meal is an opportunity to care for your mental well-being, not in a stressful way but in a nurturing way. Even small tweaks – swapping soda for water, adding an extra veggie to dinner, having a handful of nuts instead of a candy bar for a snack – can yield noticeable improvements in how you feel day-to-day. It's a wonderful, tangible example of how taking care of your body helps take care of *you* as a whole person.

Mindful Eating and Joy

For many overachievers and chronic dieters, eating has become a source of anxiety or guilt – a minefield of "shoulds" and self-judgment. Mindful eating offers a path to reclaim the simple joy of food by turning down the noise of diet rules and turning up the volume on your body's own wisdom. At its heart, mindful eating is about being present for the experience of eating, fully and without judgment. That means no more scarfing a sandwich at your desk while scrolling through emails, barely registering the taste. Instead, you give yourself permission to savor your food. You pay attention to the aroma, the texture, the flavors, and how each bite makes you feel. By focusing on the moment, eating becomes a source of pleasure and satisfaction again, not just another task to rush through. Interestingly, research has found that the opposite of mindful eating – mindless, distracted munching – is associated with overeating and even heightened anxiety. Think about when you eat in front of the TV and suddenly the entire bag of chips is gone; you were hardly aware of eating them and got little enjoyment from it. Mindful eating is the antidote to that autopilot mode. When you eat without distractions, you tend to eat more slowly and tune in to your body's signals. You may realize you're full after half a portion, or that you're satisfied with a few bites of dessert, because you actually *experienced* it. By removing the guilt and strict rules ("I shouldn't eat this, I'll regret this later") and replacing them with curiosity and acceptance, you create a healthier relationship with food. In fact, mindfulness techniques are known to reduce the shame and guilt that many people feel around eating, by promoting a non-judgmental attitude toward food choices. You learn to observe your thoughts ("I'm craving ice cream") without panic or self-criticism, and this mental shift is incredibly liberating.

One of the biggest benefits of mindful eating is that it naturally prevents overeating while increasing your satisfaction. When you eat slowly and mindfully, you give your body and brain time to register fullness and pleasure. It takes about 20 minutes for satiety signals to kick in, so if you rush through a meal in 5 minutes, you'll likely miss those signals and feel unsatisfied, even if you've eaten plenty. Mindful eating encourages you to slow down. Try taking smaller bites and chewing thoroughly, as if you were a food critic savoring each flavor note. Set down your utensil between bites. Notice the subtle sweetness of a cherry tomato or the crunch of a lettuce leaf. By engaging all your senses, you're not only extracting more joy from the food, but you're also more attuned to when you've had "just enough." Research has shown that interventions focusing on mindful eating help people become better at recognizing their fullness cues and exerting control over impulsive eating. In a review of dozens of studies, mindful eating practices led to reductions in binge eating and emotional eating, as participants learned to distinguish between true hunger and eating out of stress or boredom. Additionally, something remarkable happens when you *fully* experience your food: you often find you're satisfied with less. For example, if you slowly relish a small square of dark chocolate, noticing its rich taste, you may find that one or two pieces completely hits the spot, whereas mindlessly munching might lead you to eat an entire bar without real satisfaction. By eating mindfully, you give yourself the chance to enjoy your meals deeply, which means you won't be left hunting the pantry an hour later in search of that missing satisfaction.

Crucially, a joyful and sane approach to eating means no food is forbidden. All foods can have a place in a balanced, mindful diet. When you remove the strict "good vs. bad" labels from food, you also remove the power those forbidden foods held over you. You can finally enjoy a slice of pizza or a cookie *without* the side serving of guilt. Paradoxically, allowing all foods and truly savoring what you love can make you less likely to overindulge. There's science behind this: studies indicate that when people stop depriving themselves of certain "taboo" treats, their intense cravings for those items tend to diminish, and they don't binge on them as readily. You prove to yourself that one doughnut is not a disaster – it's just a tasty treat – and because you're not constantly dreaming of the doughnuts you "can't" have, you're free to enjoy one occasionally and move on. In one striking study, dieters who included a small dessert every day were actually more successful at maintaining weight loss than those who tried to cut out sweets entirely. The group that indulged in a bit of sweetness (like chocolate at breakfast) reported fewer cravings and ended up eating less overall, whereas the ultra-strict group eventually lost control and regained weight. The lesson is clear: you really *can* have your cake and eat it too, as long as you do so mindfully. When no food is off-limits, food loses its mystique and fear factor. A bowl of ice cream becomes just that – a bowl of ice cream – not a moral failure or a stress response. And when you choose to eat that ice cream mindfully, you're present to enjoy its creamy texture and flavor, which is far more fulfilling than mindlessly inhaling it with a side of remorse.

Ultimately, mindful eating reconnects you with the joy of food and the wisdom of your own body. It's about trust and pleasure. You trust that your body will tell you when it's hungry or had enough, and you trust yourself to listen. You also give yourself permission to enjoy eating again, as you did when you were a child and food was just yummy, not "fattening" or "allowed" or "cheating." This doesn't mean every meal becomes a slow Zen meditation – let's be realistic, sometimes you'll eat a sandwich in the car between appointments – but it does mean adopting a general attitude of presence and self-compassion with your eating. Even a few minutes of mindful eating practice a day can make a difference. You might start by committing to eat one meal or snack per day with no distractions, focusing fully on the food. You'll likely find that not only does your food taste better, but you also feel more satisfied and in tune with your needs. Over time, this practice can help break the cycle of emotional eating because you become more aware of *why* you're reaching for food – is it true hunger, or are you upset, or just bored? And if it's the latter, you can address those feelings in a more constructive way. Mindfulness fosters this clarity. By bringing joy and awareness back to the table, you transform eating from a source of stress to a source of self-care. Every meal becomes an opportunity to nourish both body and soul. You can relish your favorite foods without fear, enjoy indulgences in moderation, and feel confident that you're supporting your wellness goals at the same time. This is the essence of the Anti-Hustle Health Plan:

rejecting the grind of diet perfectionism and rediscovering a harmonious, enjoyable relationship with food. Eat to nourish yourself and enjoy it – that truly is the lazy genius way to lasting wellness.

Chapter 7

Rest and Recovery – Your Secret Weapon

Rest and Recovery – Your Secret Weapon

In a culture that glorifies grinding and pushing our limits, true strength can actually come from the opposite strategy: quality rest. Rest and recovery are the secret weapons of the "anti-hustle" health plan. They are not indulgences or signs of laziness, but essential components of fitness, sanity, and long-term success. Modern science has illuminated how giving your body and mind time to recharge boosts everything from your metabolism and mood to your muscle growth. In this chapter, we'll explore why sleep, rest days, and relaxation practices can make you stronger and happier – allowing you to achieve more by sometimes doing less.

Sleep Your Way to Strength

If there is one "lazy genius" habit to embrace for better wellness, it's sleep. Far from being wasted time, sleep is the cornerstone of your health and fitness. When you sleep, your body isn't dormant at all – it's busy repairing muscles, consolidating memories, and regulating hormones. Getting quality sleep has profound benefits for your metabolism, mood, and muscle recovery. In fact, research shows that healthy sleep helps stabilize the hormones that control appetite and weight; conversely, people who skimp on sleep often experience disrupted metabolism and weight gain. Studies have found that even a single week of cutting back on sleep can throw your hunger hormones out of balance – increasing ghrelin (which makes you feel hungry) and decreasing leptin (which signals fullness) – leading you to eat more than you otherwise would. In short, skimping on sleep can nudge your metabolism to store fat and ramp up cravings, while plenty of sleep keeps your fat-burning machinery humming. Emotionally, a good night's rest acts like a reset button – it improves mood and prevents irritability, dramatically lowering the risk of anxiety or depression. And on the physical side, sleep is when your muscles rebuild stronger. During the deep stages of sleep, your body releases growth hormone and repairs the microscopic muscle tears from your workouts, while stress hormones like cortisol dial down. This means that without enough sleep, you're short-circuiting your own strength gains and recovery.

Nothing illustrates the performance-enhancing power of sleep better than a remarkable study from Stanford University. Researchers there asked a group of college basketball players to extend their nightly sleep to around 10 hours for several weeks. The results were eye-opening: with extra sleep, the athletes sprinted faster and sharpened their shooting accuracy dramatically. On average, players' 282-foot sprint times got quicker, and their free throw and three-point shot percentages jumped by about 9%. They also reported feeling less fatigued and more upbeat during practices. The takeaway is clear – sleep is not laziness; it's a performance enhancer. By simply sleeping more, these athletes gained speed and precision that no extra hour of drills could have provided.

On the flip side, even moderate sleep deprivation can sabotage your fitness efforts. When you cut your slumber short, you're effectively draining your body's battery without fully recharging it. Studies find that a lack of sleep significantly impairs strength, endurance, and coordination, while also making exercise feel harder than it should. In one analysis, athletes who were sleep-deprived saw their aerobic endurance and muscular power plummet, and their reaction times slowed, compared to when they were well-rested. In everyday terms: after a poor night's sleep, your morning run feels more like a slog, and you're more prone to sloppy mistakes or even injuries. Chronically skimp on sleep, and you might notice you hit plateaus or start regressing despite all your hard training. The science-backed truth is that sleep is the ultimate force multiplier for fitness – it amplifies the effects of your workouts and keeps your metabolism and motivation running smoothly. Embracing this fact can be liberating for overachievers: heading to bed earlier or snagging that extra hour of sleep is not "slacking off" but a smart investment in your strength and health. Sleep scientists generally recommend that most adults get about 7 to 9 hours of sleep per night for best performance and health. It's telling that even world-class athletes strive for the high end of that range: NBA superstar LeBron James, for instance, has said he aims for 8–9 hours of sleep every night (sometimes even 10 hours) as part of his self-care routine. Think of it this way: you would never skip your nutrition or training on a regular basis and expect to improve – in the same vein, prioritizing sleep is non-negotiable for a "fit and sane" life.

Active Recovery and Relaxation

In the pursuit of fitness, more is not always better. Muscles aren't built during the workout; they're built during recovery. High achievers and elite athletes alike have discovered the value of active rest – the days or moments when you deliberately take it easy so that your body can bounce back stronger. An "active recovery" might mean taking a leisurely walk, doing some gentle yoga or stretching, or simply engaging in a light hobby that gets you moving without straining you. Unlike intense training, these easy activities increase blood circulation without adding stress, which helps flush out waste products like lactic acid and deliver fresh oxygen and nutrients to tired tissues. In effect, you're clearing out the debris from your muscles and accelerating their repair. Not only do these gentle activities help your muscles, but they also calm your mind. A stroll outdoors, for instance, can significantly lower cortisol (the primary stress hormone) and leave you feeling more serene – one study found that spending 20 to 30 minutes in nature led to a measurable drop in cortisol levels. Ever notice how a slow recovery jog or a casual bike ride the day after a tough workout can relieve soreness? That's active recovery at work – it reduces stiffness and helps you feel better faster, all while keeping your body limber.

Just as important as movement on rest days is embracing relaxation techniques that calm your nervous system. After pushing hard, your body and mind need signals that it's safe to switch into "rest and repair" mode. This is where practices like stretching, foam rolling, or even getting a massage come in. These activities ease tension in your muscles and can prevent those knots or tight spots from turning into injuries. For example, research has shown that spending a few minutes with a foam roller after a heavy workout can significantly decrease muscle soreness over the next day or two. In one study, athletes who foam-rolled after intense weightlifting felt less sore and recovered more quickly – their muscle soreness peaked in just 24 hours, whereas those who didn't foam roll were achier for 48 hours or more. Similarly, gentle yoga or a light swim can help relax overworked muscles and joints without adding strain. These methods are far from "cheating"; they are secret tools that high performers use to stay in the game longer. Top professional athletes famously invest in recovery – from regular sports massages to high-tech treatments – because they know it pays off. Even something as simple as a short nap can be a game-changer. A well-timed "fitness nap" is not laziness; it's a powerful recovery strategy. In fact, the benefits of a brief daytime nap are so real that NASA conducted a study on pilots and found that a 26-minute nap boosted performance by 34% and alertness by a whopping 54% compared to no nap. If a nap can make an astronaut or pilot more effective, imagine what it can do for a sleep-deprived office worker or a gym enthusiast.

Embracing active recovery gives you permission to relax, guilt-free, as a crucial part of your progress. Instead of feeling anxious that you're not grinding 24/7, reframe rest as productive downtime. Your muscles grow stronger in the hours you're not exercising. Your mind becomes sharper when you allow it a break from constant focus. Even elite military organizations have started to acknowledge this – for example, recent guidelines for soldiers include strategic short naps when longer sleep isn't possible, recognizing that alertness and performance depend on adequate rest. So next time your schedule calls for a rest day, remember that doing less can ultimately help you do more. By cycling intense effort with quality rest, you're setting yourself up for steady, sustainable gains without the burnout.

The Cost of Overdrive

To truly appreciate the power of rest, consider the cautionary tale of someone who learned its value the hard way. Arianna Huffington, a wildly successful media executive, once prided herself on squeezing as much work as possible into each day. Like many driven overachievers, she got by on just 3–4 hours of sleep a night, powering through red-eye flights, 5:00 am conference calls, and late-night emails. For a while, it seemed like she could do it all – but the cracks were starting to show. She later admitted she had become more irritable, reactive, and unable to savor her accomplishments during those sleep-deprived years. In April 2007, Huffington's overdrive lifestyle culminated in a dramatic wake-up call: she collapsed in her office, hitting her head on her desk and waking up in a pool of blood. Doctors found no serious disease – the diagnosis was sheer exhaustion. Her body had literally forced a shutdown after too many 18-hour days and not nearly enough recovery.

For someone so accomplished, this collapse was humbling. Huffington realized that she had been burning the candle at both ends, and it nearly broke her. In the following weeks and months, she radically changed her approach to health. She began to prioritize sleep and downtime as non-negotiable parts of her schedule. The results were nothing short of life-changing. With a full night's rest consistently under her belt, she found herself more present, clear-headed, and joyful in her daily life. Rather than falling behind, her work actually improved – she became a more effective leader, capable of making better decisions and handling challenges with a fresh mind. In fact, she later noted that her company's greatest growth spurts happened *after* she started getting enough sleep, not during the period when she was depriving herself. This revelation led Huffington to become a vocal evangelist for the power of sleep. She famously quipped that we as a society are in the midst of a "sleep deprivation crisis" and urged people to see rest not as a luxury, but as the foundation for productivity and creativity.

Huffington's story drives home a powerful lesson: relentless hustle without rest carries a heavy cost. It's not just one person's anecdote; countless professionals and athletes have faced burnout, fatigue, or injury from pushing too hard for too long. Maybe you've felt it yourself – the afternoon you nearly dozed off in a meeting after too many early mornings, or the injury that sidelined you because you never took a day off from training. The upside of hitting such a low point is the wisdom that comes after: when you learn that sometimes, doing less actually achieves more. By pulling back and caring for your basic needs – a good night's sleep, a relaxing evening off, a weekend with no work – you come back to your goals with more energy and focus. As Arianna Huffington put it, humans are not machines; we aren't built to run 24/7 with minimal downtime. If you treat yourself like a machine, eventually you will malfunction. But if you respect your biological need for rest, you unlock a sustainable path to success. Think of rest and recovery as the secret sauce that prevents breakdowns and keeps you performing at your peak for the long haul.

Building a Restful Routine

Understanding the importance of rest is one thing; actually getting good rest is another challenge, especially for busy people. The key is to build intentional rest habits into your daily life – to make restorative moments as routine as your morning coffee. Let's start with the cornerstone of recovery: better sleep habits. One of the most effective changes you can make is setting a "digital curfew" for yourself each night. Our modern devices (phones, tablets, computers) emit blue light that can trick your brain into thinking it's still daytime, suppressing the natural evening surge of melatonin – the hormone that makes you sleepy. By turning off screens at least an hour before bedtime, you allow your brain to unwind properly. Instead of scrolling or answering emails late at night, try replacing that habit with a calming ritual. Many sleep experts recommend establishing a consistent bedtime routine that signals to your body it's time to relax. This could be as simple as dimming the lights, brewing a cup of herbal tea or taking a warm shower, and reading a few pages of an enjoyable book (preferably a real book, not an e-book) each night. Over time, these cues become triggers for your mind to shift into sleep mode. As one wellness guru put it, "create a transition ritual to sleep" – for instance, Arianna Huffington's own routine involves putting away devices, taking a bath, wearing comfy pajamas, and reading poetry before lights-out. You can design your own wind-down ritual that suits your life, but the goal is the same: to slow down your racing mind and ease gently into rest. And if racing thoughts keep you up, consider journaling before bed. It can be as simple as jotting down a quick to-do list for the next day to get those nagging tasks out of your head. In one experiment, people who took five minutes to write down their upcoming tasks actually fell asleep significantly faster – on average about 9 minutes quicker – than those who wrote about tasks they had already completed. Offloading tomorrow's worries onto paper can free your mind for sleep.

Another vital strategy is to keep a consistent sleep schedule as much as possible. Our bodies thrive on regularity – going to bed and waking up around the same time each day helps regulate your internal clock, making it easier to fall asleep and wake up feeling refreshed. Consistency reinforces that natural circadian rhythm so you're sleepy when you should be and energetic when you need to be. Of course, life can throw curveballs, and sometimes late nights or early alarms happen. When they do, remember the value of power naps or brief breaks to fill the gap. If you had a rough night, a 20-minute afternoon nap can work wonders (just as NASA discovered for its pilots). Even if napping isn't feasible, simply closing your eyes at your desk for a few minutes or practicing a short relaxation exercise can help.

In fact, weaving mini-recovery moments into your daytime routine is a genius move for staying sane amid stress. One of the easiest and most effective techniques is deep breathing. It sounds almost too simple, but deliberate breathing exercises can physically lower your stress in minutes. When you're having a hectic workday, try this: push back from your computer, close your eyes, and take slow, deep breaths – inhaling through your nose and exhaling out through your mouth – for just 5 minutes. This kind of practice activates your body's parasympathetic "rest and digest" response, slowing your heart rate and calming you down. In a Stanford study, people who did a mere five minutes per day of focused breathing (such as extended exhalations or "cyclic sighing") significantly reduced their anxiety and improved their mood. Think about that – five minutes of breathing had measurable benefits on mental health and resilience. It's a perfectly portable, free tool you can use anytime, anywhere. Similarly, you might find a 5-minute guided meditation break, a brief walk around the block for fresh air, or even lying on the floor with your legs up the wall to stretch could serve as your mini recharge. The specific method matters less than the intention: give yourself permission during the day to pause and reset.

Finally, don't overlook the importance of creating an overall environment that supports rest. If possible, make your sleep space a sanctuary: a comfortable mattress and pillows, a dark, cool room, and minimal noise. Small tweaks like using blackout curtains or a white noise machine can dramatically improve the quality of your sleep. And during your waking hours, normalize the idea that taking breaks is part of being productive. For example, instead of powering through lunch at your desk, step away for even 15–20 minutes – you'll often return sharper and more efficient. Remember, restful routines are not a luxury for the lazy; they are a strategy for success. By prioritizing sleep and recovery, you're actually sharpening your edge. You'll likely find yourself with more energy at the gym, more focus at work, and a better mood throughout the day.

In summary, rest and recovery are your secret weapon in a world that often encourages the opposite. By sleeping deeply, embracing rest days and relaxed activities, and building calming rituals into your life, you're not abandoning your goals – you're fortifying yourself to reach them. The anti-hustle health plan isn't about dodging effort; it's about aligning with the way our bodies and minds truly thrive. It's a paradox that the harder you push yourself, the more you need to prioritize rest – but it's a paradox that can change your life once you embrace it. After all, the greatest victories often come not just from the workouts we do, but from the recovery that lets us come back stronger. So tonight, go ahead and turn off the lights a bit earlier, guilt-free – your body will thank you, and tomorrow you'll be ready to rise and truly shine.

Chapter 8
Purpose, Passion, and People

Wellness is not just about workouts and meal plans – it's about finding meaning and joy in the journey and sharing it with others. In this chapter, we explore how connecting your health goals to a deeper purpose, infusing your routine with passion and joy, and leaning on people around you can transform wellness from a grind into a fulfilling way of life. An "anti-hustle" health plan thrives when you know *why* you're pursuing it, genuinely enjoy the process, and build supportive relationships. Grounded in modern science and real-world stories, the sections that follow will motivate you to find your why, prioritize joy, harness the power of connection, and set healthy boundaries – so you can get fit, stay sane, and actually enjoy your life.

Find Your Why: Connecting Wellness to Purpose

Why do you want to be healthy? It's a simple question with profound implications. Identifying a personal "why" – whether it's wanting to be healthy for your kids, having energy for a passion project, or just feeling good each day – can fuel your motivation far more effectively than abstract fitness goals. When your wellness journey is tied to what truly matters to you, it becomes meaningful instead of just another task on a to-do list. For example, a parent who frames exercise as "having the energy to play with my children on the weekends" will likely find it easier to hit the park or the gym than someone exercising just to "burn calories." In psychological terms, this is the power of intrinsic motivation – doing something because it aligns with your core values or brings inner satisfaction, rather than for external rewards or pressures. Studies confirm that intrinsic, value-driven motivation is a key to sticking with healthy habits: research on exercise behavior shows that autonomous motivation (like personal enjoyment or valuing the benefits) strongly predicts long-term exercise adherence. In other words, when you have a compelling personal reason – your *why* – you're not forcing yourself to exercise; you're inspired to do it.

Groundbreaking research has even linked a strong sense of purpose to better health and longevity. In a long-term study of adults, those who described having a clear purpose in life ended up living longer than their peers over a 14-year follow-up, even after controlling for other wellness factors. Having that "reason to get up in the morning" appears to buffer against mortality risk across adulthood. In fact, psychologists have consistently found that a life purpose is an indicator of healthy aging and resilience. The benefits aren't just for seniors – purpose seems to help at any age by infusing life with direction and motivation. One fascinating finding is how purpose translates into day-to-day healthy behaviors: a recent study during the COVID-19 pandemic found that people with a stronger sense of purpose in life had fewer barriers to exercise and significantly higher intrinsic motivation to be physically active. Essentially, purpose-driven individuals *enjoyed* physical activity more and valued its benefits, which led them to move more and sit less. Instead of dragging themselves through a routine they dread, they see exercise as a means to a valued end – whether that end is being able to travel in retirement, stay mobile to enjoy hobbies, or simply live without pain. Their workouts become fuel for their mission.

Connecting wellness to your personal why can also shift your mindset from obligation to opportunity. Consider a high-achieving volunteer who hates running but loves the cause of clean water in her community. If she reframes her morning jog as training for a 5K charity run to raise money for that cause, suddenly each run has a purpose beyond just logging miles. The act of running transforms from a chore into a mission, powered by purpose. This kind of reframing taps into what behavioral scientists call "identified motivation," meaning you identify with the outcome of the behavior. Research shows that identified motives (like exercising *because* you believe in the outcome, such as health for your family or a cause) can kick-start a habit, while intrinsic enjoyment sustains it for the long run. So, if you're struggling to stick with healthy habits, step back and ask: *What truly matters to me, and how does my health support that?* You might discover that you're not really running just to run – you're running to be around for your grandkids, or to keep your creative energy high for that novel you're writing. When health ties into what genuinely matters to you, it stops being about abstract numbers on a scale or clocking arbitrary minutes on a treadmill. Instead, it becomes a means to live the life you value, which is a far more powerful motivator.

Finally, finding your why isn't a one-time thing – it can evolve. Today your why might be excelling at a passion project, and tomorrow it might be being strong enough to care for aging parents. The key is to keep your wellness journey anchored to a purpose larger than vanity or vague expectations. A sense of purpose not only propels you forward, it also provides a psychological buffer during tough times. When you encounter setbacks (and everyone does, whether in fitness or life), a strong why acts like a North Star. You can remind yourself, *"I'm doing this for that reason – that hasn't changed,"* and pick yourself back up. In sum, purpose is the heartbeat of sustainable wellness. As studies suggest, it might even help add years to your life – but more importantly, it adds life to your years, infusing each healthy choice with meaning and motivation that no superficial goal could ever match.

Joy as a Health Practice: Making Mental and Emotional Fulfillment a Priority

Wellness isn't supposed to be a miserable slog; if it is, something's gone wrong. An often-overlooked fact of health is that joy is a healing force. Making time for hobbies, creative outlets, and activities that genuinely delight you is not a luxury – it's a legitimate health practice. Think of laughter, fun, and creative absorption as vitamins for your mind and body. When you lose yourself in an activity you love – whether it's tinkering with a DIY project, walking your dog in the woods, playing guitar, or tending a garden – you enter a state that psychologists liken to "flow." In a flow state, you become fully engaged in the present moment, and worries and stressors fade into the background. Neuroscience shows that during these periods of deep engagement, stress levels drop and self-critical thoughts quiet down. In other words, doing what you love can put your brain in a restorative mode where stress hormones decrease and feel-good chemicals increase. Far from being idle goof-off time, these joyful moments can lower cortisol (the stress hormone) and boost neurotransmitters like dopamine and endorphins that elevate your mood.

Modern research resoundingly supports the health benefits of joyful hobbies. One extensive paper compiled data from over 93,000 older adults in 16 countries and found that those who had hobbies reported better overall health, greater happiness, and higher life satisfaction than those who didn't engage in leisure activities. They also had fewer symptoms of depression, suggesting that hobbies protect mental health. Notably, it didn't seem to matter *what* the hobby was – gardening, playing cards, knitting, volunteering, painting, you name it – it was the act of having a joyful pursuit that made the difference. The lead researcher of that study emphasized that the benefits of hobbies were *universal* across cultures. This means finding joy is a health strategy available to everyone, whether you're a busy executive in New York or a retiree in Tokyo. Positive emotions and fulfillment feed our well-being on a physiological level. For instance, engaging in creative arts has been shown to produce fast and measurable reductions in stress: in one experiment, adults who spent 45 minutes making art (like drawing or coloring) experienced significantly lowered cortisol levels afterward. Nearly three-quarters of participants in that study also reported feeling more confident and capable after their brief creative session. That's a remarkable outcome: under an hour of doing art not only relaxed their bodies but also uplifted their mindset.

Making joy a health practice could be as simple as swapping an hour of overtime for an hour of a beloved hobby. Consider the story of a software engineer who was perpetually burned out from long evenings at his computer. He decided to reclaim just two nights a week for something he used to love in college – playing basketball with friends. At first, he worried he was being "unproductive," but the results spoke otherwise. He laughed more in those pick-up games than he had in months, and he started sleeping better on those nights. His constant tension headaches eased. Even his colleagues noticed he seemed more upbeat on the days after basketball night. What happened here? By choosing joy – in this case, a social, active hobby – he unknowingly lowered his stress hormones and gave his mind a break, which improved his overall well-being. In fact, many such anecdotes are backed by science. Exercise can be joyful play, not just a workout: researchers note that even a trend like pickleball, often lauded for its fun factor, has mental health benefits – studies show playing pickleball reduces feelings of loneliness and increases life satisfaction by combining physical activity with social connection. And joy doesn't have to be active; creative and relaxing hobbies count too. One person might find bliss in an hour of painting or pottery, another in cooking a new recipe, another in losing themselves in a good book or playing music. These activities spark positive emotions and a sense of "flow" – and flow states have been linked to reduced anxiety and an overall sense of well-being.

To see joy as part of your health routine, it might help to actually schedule it. That's right – put "do something fun" on your calendar, just as you would a doctor's appointment or gym session. Treat it as non-negotiable self-care time. For example, one busy marketing manager began leaving work on time every Wednesday to attend a beginner's dance class. She noticed that on Thursdays, she was less stressed and even more productive at work. The dance class became her mid-week reset. Physiologically, that hour of dancing likely flooded her brain with endorphins and relieved built-up stress. Psychologically, it gave her something to look forward to and a sense of accomplishment that had nothing to do with work. This illustrates a key point: positive emotions and leisure aren't escapism; they actively repair and recharge you. Chronic stress is a major threat to health – it's linked with everything from lowered immunity to higher risk of chronic diseases – and joy is one of the most natural antidotes. When you engage in a hobby you love, your body shifts out of "fight or flight" mode. Heart rate and blood pressure can go down, muscle tension eases, and your mind clears. Over time, regularly experiencing these states can improve your baseline stress resilience.

Real-world case studies abound. In one notable example, a 53-year-old writer rediscovered her childhood passion for figure skating after decades away from the ice. She expected to just dabble, but instead found herself "reinvigorated, reinspired, reenergized" by skating again. Despite a few bumps and bruises along the way, she reported feeling happier than she had in years. It turns out science can explain her dramatic improvement: taking on a fun new challenge (or picking up an old one) in midlife stimulates the brain and body in profound ways. Learning a new skill as an adult has been shown to enhance neuroplasticity (your brain's ability to form new connections) and even improve mood and cognitive function. That skater's story ended with her performing in a local show and making new friends at the rink – proof that pursuing joy can open doors to personal growth and social connection, all while benefiting health. The takeaway for all of us is that joy is not the opposite of productivity; it is a prerequisite for sustainable wellness. When you allow yourself pleasures like hobbies and creative outlets, you're not "being lazy" – you're practicing a form of preventative medicine for your soul. So go ahead and give yourself permission to have fun. Your cortisol levels will thank you, and so will your future self.

The Power of Connection: Wellness is a Team Effort

If you want to go far, go together. Humans are profoundly social creatures, and our health is intimately connected to the quality of our relationships. In the quest for wellness, other people can be your greatest asset (or, if you're not careful, a missing ingredient). Many overachievers try to white-knuckle their health goals alone – hitting the gym solo at 5 A.M., eating a sad salad at their desk while others go out – only to find their willpower waning. But turning wellness into a *team effort* can make the process more enjoyable and dramatically boost your motivation. The science on social connection and health is eye-opening: a famous 85-year Harvard study of adult development concluded that the strongest predictor of a long, healthy life was not genes or money, but the strength of one's relationships. Participants who had supportive relationships in midlife were not only happier, but physically healthier and lived longer than those who were more isolated. Close relationships acted like a protective shield against life's slings and arrows – helping people manage stress, stay active, and even avoid lifestyle pitfalls. In contrast, loneliness and social isolation have been identified as serious health hazards. The U.S. Surgeon General recently noted that lacking social connection can increase the risk of premature death as much as smoking 15 cigarettes a day. That is a staggering comparison that puts loneliness in the same league as well-known medical risk factors. Chronic loneliness has been linked to higher rates of heart disease, stroke, and even neurodegenerative disorders; for example, older adults who are persistently lonely have a significantly higher risk (some studies say ~50% higher) of developing dementia. Clearly, *who* you spend time with (and *that* you spend time with others) is as vital to your health as not smoking or getting exercise.

The good news is that social wellness can be a joy to cultivate. Making health a group activity not only keeps loneliness at bay, but can directly improve your physical outcomes. Friends and family provide accountability ("Hey, are we still on for our evening walk?") and encouragement ("You cooked veggies for dinner – great job!") that make healthy habits easier to maintain. Something magical happens when you share the journey: workouts feel like hangouts, healthy meals become social events, and challenges feel lighter because you're not bearing them alone. For instance, consider joining a walking group or starting a weekly healthy potluck with friends. The simple act of walking and chatting with a friend can turn exercise into an hour you genuinely look forward to. By pairing a positive social experience with physical activity, you reinforce the habit on multiple levels – psychologically (it's fun, so you want to do it), and practically (someone else is counting on you to show up).

Research backs this up. One classic study found that married couples who joined a fitness program together had dramatically better adherence after 12 months compared to married individuals who joined alone: the pair who worked out together had higher attendance and a far lower dropout rate (only about 6% of the couples quit, versus 43% of the solo participants). The researchers noted that spousal support – having someone at home encouraging you and sharing the routine – made all the difference in sticking with the program. While that study focused on spouses, the principle extends to any workout buddy or group. Mutual support and a dash of friendly peer pressure can nudge you out the door on the days your motivation lags.

Social connection also introduces an element of fun and play that is hard to replicate alone. Think about it: a solo gym session might check the box, but a Zumba class or pickup soccer game with friends can lift your spirits while you sweat. Laughing burns calories too! Turning healthy activities into social outings – like biking with a buddy on weekends or hosting a healthy recipe swap night – helps you associate wellness with positive emotions. Instead of viewing your health habits as a solo chore, they become part of your *social life*. During the pandemic lockdowns, many people realized how much easier it was to take a daily walk when it doubled as a chance to connect with family or neighbors (even if just waving from across the street). Post-pandemic, the rise of group activities like community fun runs, group meditation sessions, or online fitness challenges shows that we crave doing things together. Even introverts benefit from having a support system, if only a small one. You might prefer one-on-one hikes with a close friend rather than a big group class – what matters is that you feel connected.

Aside from motivation, friends and family can offer tangible help and new perspectives. You can swap healthy recipes, share tips, or even team up on goals (like training for a charity walk as a team). If you struggle with a particular aspect of wellness, consider recruiting a friend to do it with you. Not a morning person? Find a colleague who also wants a morning jog, and you can be sunrise accountability partners. Hate cooking alone? Turn Sunday meal prep into a family affair – put on some music and give everyone a task. These moments strengthen your relationships, which in turn reinforces your commitment to health. It's a virtuous cycle: strong relationships make you healthier, and pursuing health together can make your relationships stronger. One study even suggested that eating together frequently is associated with greater life satisfaction and happiness – a reminder that sharing healthy meals can nourish both body and soul. The bottom line: wellness does not have to be a lonely road. In fact, it's often the *community* you build around healthy living that keeps you going when the road gets rough. By leaning on others and letting them lean on you, you gain motivation, enjoyment, and a sense of belonging – all powerful boosts to your overall well-being.

Boundaries and Balance: Saying "No" to Burnout, "Yes" to Self-Care

For the overachievers and people-pleasers of the world, this may be the hardest lesson of all: taking care of yourself often means saying "no" to others. If you are used to saying "yes" to every request – staying late at work, helping everyone who asks, filling every minute with obligations – your wellness will pay the price. In the long run, you simply *cannot pour from an empty cup*. Setting boundaries on your time and energy isn't selfish; it's essential. This section is your permission slip to protect your well-being by drawing lines where needed, so you don't burn out.

Burnout has become so common that the World Health Organization now recognizes it as an occupational phenomenon, resulting from chronic workplace stress. It's no surprise that those most at risk are often the high-achieving, always-on individuals who never learned to hit the brakes. The health consequences of an unbounded, always-yes lifestyle are severe. Working excessively long hours, for instance, has been linked to higher risks of serious illness. A global study by the WHO found that regularly putting in 55 or more hours per week was associated with a 35% higher risk of stroke and a 17% higher risk of dying from heart disease, compared to a standard 35–40 hour workweek. In the study's words, "Working 55 hours or more per week is a *serious health hazard*". Yet many overachievers do just that, week after week, thinking they are being responsible or productive, when in reality they are slowly undermining their health. Beyond the physical toll, never saying no takes a huge mental toll. You might start to notice signs of *poor boundaries* in your life: feeling constantly taken advantage of, resenting commitments you've made, being exhausted, anxious, or inexplicably sad about your schedule. These feelings of resentment and depletion are not just mood swings – they are red flags that you are overextended and headed for burnout.

Psychologists define boundaries as the limits and rules we set for ourselves in relationships and activities, which protect our well-being. Without clear boundaries, we give others (or our work) free rein to dictate our lives, and we end up stretched thin. The result is often that subtle, but powerful, state of burnout – characterized by exhaustion, cynicism, and a sense of reduced efficacy. Burnout often looks like chronic fatigue, irritability, lack of joy in things you used to enjoy, and even physical symptoms like headaches or insomnia. It can mimic depression and anxiety. Crucially, burnout is frequently linked to saying "yes" too often – taking on more than you reasonably can handle. People who burn out often report that work (or caregiving, or whatever domain) took over their life, crowding out rest, hobbies, and social time. This is where boundaries come in as a powerful antidote. *Establishing boundaries can prevent and even heal burnout by restoring balance to your life.* Think of boundaries as the guardrails on a winding mountain road – without them, it's easy to veer off into dangerous territory. With them, you have guidance and safety.

How do you start setting boundaries, especially if you're not used to it? First, remind yourself (often and emphatically) that self-care is not selfish. One therapist put it this way: "Paying attention to your needs is self-care. And like putting on your oxygen mask first on an airplane, you'll have more energy for others if you apply it to yourself first". This means that saying no to an extra project or turning down a social invitation when you're exhausted is actually an act of kindness – both to yourself and ultimately to the people you care about, because it helps ensure you'll be healthy and present in the long run. Next, get comfortable with the word "no" itself. This can be challenging for chronic yes-sayers. Start small if needed: practice declining something minor, or set a small boundary like not answering work emails after 8 PM. Notice the world doesn't end when you do this! In fact, many times people will respect you *more* when they see you respect yourself. Communicating boundaries can be done gracefully: you can say "I'd love to help, but I have too much on my plate right now," or "I need to decline so I can focus on some personal commitments." No need to over-justify or apologize profusely. Setting a boundary is simply stating what you need – a basic right in any healthy relationship or workplace.

It also helps to carve out non-negotiable personal time in your schedule. Literally block it off on your calendar as you would an important meeting. This might be 30 minutes each morning to stretch and have coffee in peace, or a commitment that you don't work on Sundays, or an agreement with your partner that Wednesday evenings are your time to hit the gym or read alone. When others inevitably encroach ("Could you handle this by tomorrow morning?" or "Can we schedule this call Wednesday night?"), having that time marked off in your mind allows you to confidently respond, "I'm not available then." Remember, *every time you say yes to something, you are saying no to something else.* If you say yes to a late meeting, you might be saying no to your workout or family dinner. Boundaries help you be conscious of those trade-offs so you choose wisely. Protecting time for sleep, exercise, meal prep, and relaxation isn't lazy – it's how top performers in any field avoid burnout and maintain high output. As counterintuitive as it seems, setting limits on work can actually improve your work. The WHO study even noted that companies benefit from capping excessive hours because well-rested workers are more productive. So by drawing that line, you're not only safeguarding your health, you may also be enhancing your effectiveness in the long run.

Finally, let's address the guilt that often comes with boundary-setting. You might worry that you're letting people down or not living up to expectations. It can help to reframe boundaries as healthy discipline rather than selfishness. Just as an athlete must discipline their training and rest to avoid injury, you are disciplining your life to avoid burnout. When you set a boundary like "no work emails after dinner" or "Sunday is family time," you are honoring your values and needs. Communicate this if appropriate – for example, tell your team, "I've found I need to unplug on the weekends to recharge; I'll respond to any pending items first thing Monday." Reasonable people will understand (and those who don't, well, that's telling). Over time, the guilt lessens as you experience the positive results: you start feeling less stressed, more in control, and more *present.* Indeed, clinicians note that when people establish better work-life boundaries, they often reclaim the energy to be present in their relationships and re-engage with hobbies or sources of joy. In essence, saying "no" to constant commitments is saying "yes" to a healthier, saner you.

In practice, here are a few boundary-setting tips: Identify your top values and priorities (family, health, creativity, etc.) – use those as a guide for what deserves your time. Get comfortable with the idea that you don't have to do it all; sometimes "good enough" truly is good enough. Start implementing small boundaries (like a fixed bedtime or a daily lunch break away from your desk) and gradually move to bigger ones (like declining a promotion that would destroy your work-life balance, or stepping back from a volunteer role that no longer fits). And remember, every time you set a healthy boundary, you serve as a role model to others that well-being matters. Far from disappointing people, you might inspire them to take better care of themselves too.

Conclusion: Your Wellness, Your Way (with Purpose, Passion, People, and Peace)

As we conclude this chapter on "Purpose, Passion, and People," take a moment to envision what an *anti-hustle* approach to wellness could look like in your life. Imagine pursuing health not as a frantic race, but as a joyful journey fueled by what matters most to you. You wake up with a sense of purpose, knowing why you care about your health. You build passion and joy into your routine – perhaps a morning stretch while listening to your favorite music or an evening hobby that lights you up. You lean on people – partnering up for workouts, sharing laughter at healthy dinners, and drawing strength from a community that supports your goals. And you maintain balance by setting boundaries, confidently saying no when you must, and giving yourself permission to rest. This isn't a fantasy; it's a very attainable reality, backed by science and lived out by countless individuals who traded the burnout cycle for a more sustainable rhythm. By finding your why, prioritizing joy, embracing connection, and respecting your own limits, you can get fit and stay sane – and yes, *actually enjoy your life* – as a true lazy genius of wellness. Each positive choice, no matter how small, is an investment in the vibrant, meaningful life you deserve. Now go forth and craft your Anti-Hustle Health Plan – one purposeful, passionate, people-filled, and well-balanced day at a time.

Chapter 9

Mindset Mastery for Sustainable Wellness

The journey to lasting wellness isn't just about finding the right diet or exercise plan – it's about cultivating a mindset that makes healthy living feel sustainable and even enjoyable. Our minds can be our biggest allies or our worst saboteurs. Many overachievers and burned-out individuals approach wellness with the same all-or-nothing intensity that drives their work, only to find themselves frustrated. In this chapter, we focus on mastering the mindset behind sustainable wellness. That means embracing progress over perfection, learning to bounce back from setbacks with resilience and self-compassion, freeing ourselves from toxic comparisons, and shifting our very identity to align with a balanced, anti-hustle approach to health. These mental shifts are the true "lazy genius" strategies that enable you to get fit, stay sane, and actually enjoy your life in the long run. Let's dive into each of these key elements of mindset mastery.

Progress Over Perfection

Even a brisk 15-minute daily walk can yield significant health benefits. Research shows a 15-minute fast walk each day can cut risk of death by nearly 20% – a powerful reminder that small consistent actions matter more than occasional heroic efforts.

One of the most common mindset traps in wellness (and life) is perfectionism. It's the voice that tells you that if you can't do something perfectly, you shouldn't bother doing it at all. We've all been there: perhaps you set a goal to work out an hour every day, eat an impeccably clean diet, or meditate every morning at 5 AM. Then reality intervenes – a day gets busy or you feel tired – and you miss one workout or grab some fast food. The perfectionist impulse declares the whole plan ruined, leading many to quit entirely. This all-or-nothing thinking is a recipe for failure. In truth, doing *something* usually beats doing nothing. A 15-minute walk on a busy day absolutely counts, both for your health and for maintaining momentum. Those small wins add up. In fact, research confirms that even very short bouts of activity can have tangible benefits: for example, a quick 15-minute walk can curb cravings for sweets and reduce stress-eating, on top of the longer-term health benefits. The key is to celebrate these small wins instead of dismissing them.

Perfectionism doesn't just steal the joy from our efforts – it can outright prevent progress. Psychologists often remind us that *"perfect is the enemy of good,"* a saying attributed to Voltaire. Facebook's COO Sheryl Sandberg echoed this idea with a sign in her office that reads, "Done is better than perfect." As Sandberg explains, aiming for impossibly high standards often leads to frustration and paralysis. In other words, if you insist on a perfect plan or perfect performance, you may end up never starting or finishing anything. Research bears this out: those with strong perfectionist tendencies often struggle with procrastination and burnout. They delay tasks out of fear of failure, or obsess over tiny details. One Harvard article noted that perfectionists are frequently *"reluctant to start new projects or activities out of fear of failure"* and that their quest for perfection can cause tasks to take much longer than needed. Even more concerning, chronic perfectionism has been linked to higher rates of stress, anxiety, and depression. In short, the perfectionism trap doesn't lead to superior results – it leads to stagnation and misery.

So, how do we escape this trap? By consciously adopting a progress over perfection mindset. This means recognizing that consistent good efforts will beat sporadic perfect ones. It means telling yourself that it's better to do a *pretty good* workout today than to plan a "perfect" workout and never do it. It means being proud of choosing a side salad instead of fries most of the time, rather than feeling like a failure forever eating fries at all. Consider the story of Allison, a marketing executive and mother of two who used to believe that if she couldn't go hard at the gym for an hour, it wasn't worth exercising. With her schedule, that meant she rarely exercised at all. After hitting a wall with her energy levels, Allison tried a different approach: she walked for 15–20 minutes in her neighborhood after work, and did a quick 10-minute yoga or stretching routine before bed. These sessions were far from the "ideal" 90-minute intense workouts she had in mind, but she did them consistently – almost every day – because they actually fit her life. After a few months, Allison noticed she was more flexible, slept better, and had shed a few pounds. More importantly, she felt proud and motivated. *"Once I saw those small improvements,"* she says, *"I realized how empowering good enough can be. I wasn't failing; I was building."* Her story illustrates a powerful truth: small daily actions compound over time. They create momentum and confidence. Over a year, Allison's tiny routines added up to well over a hundred hours of movement – far more than she would have gotten aiming for perfection and quitting early.

Indeed, behavioral science supports the power of focusing on progress. Teresa Amabile's research at Harvard on the *"progress principle"* finds that making even incremental progress on meaningful goals boosts our motivation and mood. In the context of wellness, this means you should give yourself credit for every healthy choice, no matter how minor. Did you squeeze in a quick stretch between Zoom meetings? Celebrate it. Chose water over soda today? That's a win. Over time, these victories build a positive feedback loop: you feel good about doing something, which makes you more likely to continue. By contrast, if you fixate on perfection, you're setting yourself up to feel like a failure (and then abandon your efforts) at the first slip. Consistency is far more important than perfection for sustainable wellness. As one wise saying goes, *"An imperfect workout you actually do is better than the perfect workout you don't."* Progress over perfection is about giving yourself permission to be human – to do your best on each day, recognizing that best will vary – and knowing that good enough really is good enough to get you to your goals.

To reinforce this mindset, it helps to look at examples of success through consistency. One famous illustration comes from the tech world: early Facebook teams embraced the mantra *"Done is better than perfect"*, meaning it was more valuable to make steady improvements than to hold back until something could be released flawlessly. In fitness and health, we see similar stories. For instance, many participants of the popular

Couch to 5K running program start out barely able to jog for one minute, but by focusing on gradual progress – just doing a bit more each week – they end up running a full 5K after two months. Their success comes not from any single perfect run, but from persistent, "good enough" runs strung together. Or consider legendary comedian Jerry Seinfeld's productivity secret: he would mark an "X" on a calendar for each day he wrote new jokes, telling aspiring writers to simply "not break the chain." The brilliance of that approach is its focus on consistency over brilliance – some days he wrote mediocre jokes, some days great ones, but by writing daily he amassed an outstanding body of work. The lesson for our wellness journey is clear: doing something regularly, even imperfectly, leads to big results over time. If you keep showing up – taking that walk, choosing a healthier meal, going to bed earlier – you will be amazed at where you are in a year compared to the stop-start cycle of perfectionism.

In practical terms, embracing progress over perfection means being kinder to yourself and adjusting your standards. Set achievable micro-goals: if you plan to exercise 5 days a week and only manage 3, view that as 3 days of success (not 2 days of failure). If you planned to eat five servings of veggies and only got two, applaud yourself for those two and try for more tomorrow. By shifting your focus to progress and small wins, you keep yourself in the game. You'll stay motivated because you're *acknowledging your efforts*, not just your shortcomings. This mindset frees you from the weight of unrealistic expectations and helps you enjoy the process. As a result, you'll find that healthy habits start to feel less like a chore and more like a series of positive choices you want to make. Progress over perfection isn't about lowering your standards or abandoning ambition – it's about trading impossible standards for sustainable ones. It's a commitment to growth, one day at a time, which is ultimately far more effective (and rewarding) than chasing an ever-moving bar of "perfect."

Bouncing Back from Setbacks

No matter how committed or consistent you are, setbacks are inevitable on any wellness journey. Life will throw curveballs: an illness or injury might knock you off your exercise routine, a crunch period at work might disrupt your meal planning, or you might simply hit a motivation slump where the couch looks far more inviting than the gym. The difference between those who ultimately succeed in their wellness goals and those who give up isn't that the successful ones never slip up – it's that they recover and restart when they do. In this section, we'll prepare for those inevitable obstacles and discuss how to bounce back with resilience, *without* falling into guilt or all-or-nothing thinking. Remember, resilience – the ability to keep going after a setback – is more important in the long run than never slipping up in the first place.

First, it's crucial to normalize setbacks. They happen to everyone, even the most disciplined individuals. Olympians have rest days and off-seasons; wellness gurus admit to days when they eat junk or skip workouts. Rather than viewing a setback as a catastrophic failure, try to see it as a *temporary detour*. One bad week doesn't erase the progress you've made. What matters most is what you do next. Adopting this perspective takes the pressure off: if you expect that occasional lapses will occur, you can greet them with a plan instead of panic. For example, David, a 45-

year-old sales manager, had built a solid habit of jogging three mornings a week. When a busy season forced him to travel and he went two weeks without running, old perfectionist thoughts crept in: *"You've blown it – might as well forget the whole thing."* But David caught himself and reframed the situation. Two weeks off didn't mean all fitness was lost; it simply meant it was time to lace up his shoes again. He resumed with a lighter routine (shorter, slower runs to get back into rhythm) and was careful not to punish himself mentally. Within another two weeks, he was right back on track. David's story underscores a key point: a lapse isn't a collapse. Missing some workouts or eating poorly for a spell doesn't define you or your journey – how you respond does.

One of the most effective strategies for bouncing back is to revisit your "why." When motivation wanes or you feel discouraged by a setback, reconnect with the deeper reason you started your wellness journey. Maybe your "why" is to have more energy to play with your kids, to reduce stress and anxiety, to improve your long-term health and avoid the illnesses that run in your family, or simply to feel more confident and alive in your body. Reminding yourself of this core purpose can reignite your drive. For instance, when *Maria* finds herself in a slump and skipping her evening walks, she sits down and writes in her journal about why she began prioritizing her health – she pictures being around to dance at her daughter's future wedding, and remembers how much calmer she feels after walking. That emotional reconnection provides the spark to get moving again. Your reasons are your fuel; when the tank is low, go back to the source and refill it.

Another powerful tool for overcoming setbacks is self-compassion. This might sound counterintuitive to those used to tough self-criticism, but research shows that being kind to yourself after a slip-up actually increases the likelihood of getting back on track, whereas guilt and self-shaming often make things worse. Consider a striking study: dieters in an experiment were all given a doughnut to eat (so, essentially, induced to break their diet). But only some were then given a compassionate message ("Everyone eats unhealthy foods sometimes – you haven't blown anything, so don't be hard on yourself"). Those who received this small dose of kindness ate significantly less candy in a subsequent taste test, while those who felt guilty about the doughnut ended up eating more candy, turning a minor lapse into a larger one. In other words, forgiving themselves helped people stop a slip from spiraling into a binge. As one of the study authors put it, *"self-compassion is the missing ingredient in every diet and weight-loss plan".* The logic is simple: when you respond to a setback with harsh self-criticism (*"I'm so weak; I failed again"*), you feel demoralized and ashamed – emotions that often drive comfort eating or giving up. But when you respond with kindness (*"I'm human; it's okay. I can learn from this and resume my plan"*), you create a mental space to regroup without the extra burden of shame. Self-compassion isn't about letting yourself off the hook indefinitely; it's about encouraging yourself the way you would a good friend – with understanding and support to help you move forward.

Practicing self-compassion can be as straightforward as noticing your self-talk and deliberately shifting its tone. Instead of *"I have no discipline, I blew my routine,"* tell yourself, *"I've been working hard, and this week was tough.*

It's normal to slip. I can start fresh tomorrow." Some people find it helpful to imagine what they'd say to a friend or what a good coach would say to them – usually we find those words are much gentler and more constructive. Research in health psychology consistently finds that shame and guilt tend to sap motivation, whereas a self-compassionate attitude boosts it. By being kind to yourself, you are more likely to stay motivated to do the healthy behavior again, rather than hiding from it out of self-loathing.

Besides self-compassion, another tactic for bouncing back is to scale back to easier tasks until you regain confidence and momentum. When you've fallen off the wagon, the hardest part is often overcoming inertia. You might feel overwhelmed thinking about doing the full intensity of what you were doing before. So, make it easier. If you haven't exercised in a month, maybe don't jump straight into a full hour spin class – start with a 10-minute gentle bike ride or a short walk. If cooking healthy meals feels like too much right now, consider buying pre-cut veggies or healthy ready-made options to ease back into better eating. The idea is to create quick wins for yourself to rebuild the habit. For example, Nina, who struggled with depression over the winter and stopped going to the gym, gave herself permission to do just one set of exercises at home to start. It seemed almost too easy – exactly the point. After completing one set, she felt a small sense of accomplishment, which often led her to do a second set. Within two weeks, she felt ready to return to the gym for short sessions. This approach of taking tiny steps is backed by behavior science: it lowers the barrier to action. You're "mastering the art of showing up," as habit expert James Clear says. Once you're showing up again, even in a small way, you can gradually increase the challenge. The crucial thing is that you're moving forward again, proving to yourself that the setback was just a pause, not a full stop.

Let's consolidate these strategies. When you find yourself off track, remember the Three Rs: Reconnect, Reframe, Restart. Reconnect to your why – the deeper motivation that gives your journey meaning. Reframe the setback with self-compassion – talk to yourself like a friend and ditch the guilt. Then Restart with a small, manageable action to get momentum back. You might even write these down somewhere visible as a personal action plan for future slumps. Embracing this resilient mindset means that instead of a downward spiral, your setbacks will become springboards. Every time you bounce back, you strengthen the habit of not quitting. You learn that *you are the kind of person who keeps going.* Over time, this builds an unshakable confidence. You come to trust that no matter how many times you slip, you will never let it turn into permanent failure. And that might be the most important healthy habit of all.

The Comparison Detox

Nothing can sap the enjoyment out of your wellness journey quite like comparison – especially in the age of social media, where we're inundated with images of other people's highlight reels. You might find yourself scrolling through Instagram or TikTok and seeing fitness influencers with chiseled abs, or reading about a colleague's marathon training, and suddenly your own perfectly good efforts feel inadequate. But comparing your progress or body or routine to someone else's is not only unfair – it's downright toxic to motivation. In this section, we'll explore why social comparison is a dead-end and how to free yourself from it. Consider this your guide to a Comparison Detox: a deliberate process of focusing on *your own journey* and tuning out the noise of others' results.

The problem with comparison is that we tend to compare our *behind-the-scenes* with other people's *highlight reels*. Social media makes this worse by providing a constant stream of curated, idealized content. People typically showcase their best moments: the longest run, the healthiest salad, the post-workout selfie when they're feeling great. We don't see the struggles, the bad days, the Photoshop or filters. Yet our brains mistakenly stack our reality against that illusion. It's no wonder that study after study has found heavy social media use is linked to lower self-esteem and body satisfaction. For example, research on Instagram usage shows that the more time young women spend on the platform, the more their body image and self-worth tend to suffer. Psychologists attribute this largely to upward social comparisons – we constantly see people who seem to be doing "better" than us, which breeds feelings of inadequacy. Even beyond body image, social comparison can give a skewed sense of what "normal" progress looks like. If your feed is full of friends running ultra-marathons or doing intense 5 AM bootcamps, you might feel that *everyone* is super fit and dedicated except you. But that's an illusion. You might be comparing yourself to the top 1% of enthusiasts and ignoring the fact that maybe those folks don't have the same circumstances or priorities as you. As the old saying goes, *"Comparison is the thief of joy."* It can steal the pride you should rightfully feel about your own improvements, and it can drain your motivation by making you feel perpetually "behind" or "not good enough."

One powerful step in the Comparison Detox is to curate your inputs. If certain social media accounts make you feel lousy about yourself, mute or unfollow them. You have control over what you consume. Consider replacing the fitspo influencers with more down-to-earth, body-positive voices – or taking a break from the scroll entirely. A tip from psychologists: try a social media fast for a week and note how you feel. Many people report a huge boost in mood and self-focus when they're not constantly checking others' lives. In place of watching others, use that time to invest in *your* wellness (or any hobby or rest you enjoy). For example, one of our readers, Joanne, realized that every morning she was spending 20 minutes in bed looking at a fitness instructor's posts and feeling demoralized that she wasn't exercising at dawn with a six-pack. She decided to unfollow that account and instead used those 20 minutes to do a short gentle yoga routine in her living room. *"It's ironic,"* she laughs, *"I used to watch someone else work out and feel bad. Now I actually do a little workout and feel great!"* By removing the source of unhealthy comparison, Joanne was able to focus on herself and make positive changes.

Another crucial element is to measure your progress against your own past self, not anybody else. This means shifting the frame: the only person you should compare yourself to is the *old you*. Are you doing something today you couldn't do three months ago? Are you a bit stronger, more flexible, more energetic, or perhaps kinder to yourself than you used to be? Those are the comparisons that matter. If last year you were winded after one flight of stairs and today you can take three flights with ease, that's a huge win – regardless of whether your coworker runs 10Ks on the weekend. If you used to be chronically sleep-deprived and now you've established a healthy sleep routine, that improvement is golden – no matter what some biohacking blogger's routine looks like. When you focus on your personal growth, you transform wellness from a competition into a personal journey. This mindset is not only more enjoyable, it's also more sustainable. You're less likely to give up because someone else seems "ahead"; instead, you're motivated by seeing how far *you've* come.

It might help to literally document your own progress. Keep a simple journal or use an app to log small milestones: the first time you could hold a plank for a minute, the fact that you've been consistently eating breakfast instead of just coffee, or how your mood has improved since you started evening walks. These notes become evidence of your trajectory. On days when you feel tempted to compare, glance at your own progress log to remind yourself of your upward trend. Tom, a 50-year-old who started weight training for the first time last year, found this very effective. He was initially embarrassed at the gym, lifting the lightest weights while seeing others heft heavy barbells. But he kept a notebook where he recorded his own weights and reps. Over months, he saw his numbers climb from very modest beginnings to actually quite respectable levels. This concrete proof of improvement gave him pride. *"I'm twice as strong as I was when I began,"* he says, *"Who cares if I'm still lifting less than the guy next to me? I'm way stronger than the old me."* Tom's attitude is a shining example of the comparison detox in action – he broke free from social comparison by focusing on personal comparison, and in doing so, he found more enjoyment in the process. He could actually celebrate his wins instead of feeling overshadowed.

Also, remember that everyone's circumstances and bodies are different. Your colleague who hits the gym at 6 AM might not have the family or commute responsibilities you do. The friend with the sculpted physique might be 15 years younger or genetically predisposed to build muscle faster. When you catch yourself idolizing or envying someone's progress, pause and remind yourself: *Their journey is not my journey.* You are writing your own unique wellness story, tailored to your life. The only standards that matter are the ones that serve your well-being. This doesn't mean you can't learn from others or be inspired by them – you absolutely can. But there's a difference between inspiration and comparison. Inspiration says, "Wow, they can do it – maybe I can find a way to do something meaningful for me." Comparison, on the other hand, says, "They're doing better than me – I'm not good enough." If a certain input consistently leads you to that negative space, it's time to cut it out. If it sparks a positive idea or motivation in you, great – use it as fuel, then turn your focus back to yourself.

In summary, undertake a Comparison Detox by cleansing your social feeds and habits of unhelpful comparisons, and by redirecting your attention to your own progress and goals. You'll likely find that when the "noise" of what others are doing quiets down, you can hear your own voice and intuition much more clearly. That inner voice can guide you toward what genuinely works for you, which might be very different from what works for someone else. And when you free yourself from chasing others' standards, you reclaim the joy in your journey. You start to appreciate the intrinsic rewards of wellness – how it makes you feel, how it enriches your life – rather than constantly grading yourself against external benchmarks. This mental shift can make *all* the difference in staying motivated and satisfied along the way.

Identity and Habit Shift

Up until now, we've talked about mindset changes you can adopt – valuing progress, practicing resilience, ignoring comparisons. In this final section, we delve into a deeper transformation: changing the way you see yourself. Lasting wellness isn't just about what you do; it's about who you become. When healthy habits move from being merely tasks on your to-do list to becoming an integrated part of your identity, they get infinitely easier to maintain. We'll explore how shifting your identity and leveraging the science of habit formation can lock in sustainable wellness without constant willpower or "hustle." This is about becoming someone who lives the anti-hustle health plan as a *way of being* – "I am someone who takes care of myself in a balanced, sane manner" – rather than viewing wellness as a temporary project or a burdensome duty.

Behavioral scientists have found that our self-identity plays a huge role in our actions. We tend to act in alignment with the person we believe ourselves to be (or the person we want to be). One remarkable study demonstrated this with something as simple as voting. Researchers discovered that people who were encouraged to think of themselves as "voters" were significantly more likely to actually go vote than those who were just urged to "go vote." In one experiment during a U.S. election, 82% of those asked about *"voting"* turned out to vote, but 96% of those asked about *"being a voter"* turned out. The only difference was the framing that invoked their identity. Being *a voter* is an identity; voting is an action. When people adopted the identity ("I am a voter"), they behaved consistently with that identity and voted in huge numbers. This principle applies to health behaviors too. If you start to see yourself as *"a healthy person"* or *"someone who prioritizes wellness,"* your daily choices will begin to line up with that self-image. You might unconsciously start taking the stairs more or choosing water over soda, because *that's what a healthy person would do.* It becomes natural, even satisfying, to act out your identity.

How do you cultivate this kind of identity shift? Start by choosing a simple, empowering identity statement that resonates with you. It could be *"I am someone who moves my body every day,"* or *"I am a person who cares for my mental and physical health,"* or even as straightforward as *"I am an active, balanced individual."* Don't worry if it feels a bit aspirational at first – that's okay. You are essentially planting a flag in the ground for who you want to become, and then letting your habits steadily catch up to that vision. The next step is to reinforce that identity with tiny, consistent habits (much like evidence that accumulates in favor of your new identity). Think of each small action as casting a "vote" for the type of person you want to be, as author James Clear puts it. For instance, each time you choose a nourishing meal, you are casting a vote for *"I am a healthy eater."* Each night you get to bed on time, you reinforce *"I am someone who respects my need for rest."* None of these actions have to be big or perfect –

consistency matters far more. Over time, the accumulation of these "votes" gives you proof of your new identity. It's not empty affirmation; you'll have tangible evidence in your own life.

Habit science offers some practical techniques to help lock in these identity-based habits. One golden rule is to start small – absurdly small, if necessary – to ensure consistency. Remember our earlier discussion of showing up and the story of the man who lost over 100 pounds by committing to just 5 minutes at the gym each day? He wasn't even allowed to stay longer than five minutes initially. To outsiders it seemed laughable – what can you accomplish in 5 minutes? – but what he *was* accomplishing was becoming the type of person who never misses workouts. He "mastered the art of showing up". Once the habit (and by extension the identity of being a regular exerciser) was established, it was easy to expand the activity. You can apply this in your own life. If you want to adopt the identity of "someone who takes daily walks," begin with a ridiculously easy walk around the block each day. If you aspire to be a meditator, start with just one minute of meditation each morning. These tiny habits may seem insignificant, but they are the seed that grows into a stable routine. Crucially, they are so small that you won't resist doing them – you don't need extreme motivation to floss one tooth or do two push-ups. Yet doing them consistently changes how you think about yourself: *"Look, I'm doing this every day – I'm keeping a promise to myself."* That feeling is immensely powerful.

Neuroscience tells us that habits form as we repeat behaviors in consistent contexts – essentially we're rewiring our brain pathways so that certain actions become automatic responses. In fact, about 43% of our daily actions are habitual, done without deliberate decision-making. This can be encouraging when it comes to wellness: imagine nearly half of your healthy behaviors happening on autopilot because they're just part of who you are! To get there, though, you need to persist in the early stages of habit formation until the behavior sticks. This is where identity helps immensely. If you're just forcing yourself to go through the motions of a habit you don't identify with (say, running every morning but internally thinking "Ugh, I hate running, I'm not a runner"), it will always feel like a battle. But if you shift your mindset to *"I'm a runner"* – even if you have to say it before it fully feels true – then each run isn't just a chore, it's an act of affirming who you are. That alignment between your identity and your actions removes a lot of the internal resistance. You're not battling yourself to do the healthy thing; the healthy thing is an expression of yourself.

Real-world case studies show the effectiveness of identity shifts. Consider Carla, who had struggled for years to stick to any exercise routine. She would sign up for programs and quit by week three. When she learned about identity-based habits, she decided to experiment. Carla loved the idea of being the kind of person who enjoys nature and activity, so she started telling herself, *"I'm an outdoorsy, active person."* It sounded almost comical at first – this was someone who usually preferred TV on the couch. But she began with tiny steps to "prove" it: every morning, she would step outside for just 5 minutes with her coffee, simply to reinforce *"I get outdoors every day."* On some days, that five minutes turned into a short walk when she felt up for it. She also joined a weekend hiking group for beginners, figuring that's what an "outdoorsy" person might do. Fast forward six months: Carla hikes nearly every weekend, walks most evenings, and has a circle of active friends. She credits the identity shift for the change: *"Once I started seeing myself differently, my behaviors followed. I'm not forcing myself to exercise now – it's just part of my life because that's who I am."* What Carla experienced is backed by research and countless anecdotal reports: when wellness actions become part of your identity, they feel natural and sustainable, not like a constant willpower struggle.

Along with identity, make use of habit cues and routines to cement behaviors. For example, tie a new healthy habit to an existing routine (this is known as habit stacking). If you want to adopt the identity "I am someone who takes care of my mental health," and you decide that daily meditation is one habit to support that, you could stack it onto something you already do: *"After I brush my teeth in the morning, I will sit and meditate for 2 minutes."* The tooth brushing is an existing cue; the 2-minute meditation is the tiny habit; together they reinforce the identity of a calm, mindful person. The more you repeat that sequence, the more automatic it becomes. Soon, skipping it will feel off – just like forgetting to brush your teeth would feel wrong. This automation is the holy grail because it means you don't have to debate with yourself each day about the healthy behavior; it just happens. That frees up mental energy and reduces the risk of falling off the routine when life gets busy.

Finally, be patient and celebrate the evolution of your identity. It's okay if at first you feel like you're "faking it till you make it." In truth, you are simply training your brain to embrace a new self-image. Over time, there will be a tipping point where you genuinely feel, *"This is me."* You'll know it has happened when skipping a workout or eating very unhealthily starts to feel inconsistent with your identity – not in an oppressive guilt way, but more like *"This just isn't like me, and I prefer to get back to my usual habits."* At that stage, you have successfully made wellness *part of who you are.* Healthy choices become almost second nature, requiring much less conscious effort to maintain. You'll have shifted from *doing* healthy things to *being* a healthy (and balanced) person.

To wrap up, mindset mastery for sustainable wellness is about these profound yet achievable shifts in how you think about progress, setbacks, comparisons, and yourself. By prioritizing progress over perfection, you give yourself permission to be imperfect and thus remain consistent. By learning to bounce back with resilience and self-compassion, you ensure that obstacles become learning experiences rather than dead-ends. By detoxing from comparisons, you reclaim joy and motivation that come from within, measured on your own terms. And by shifting your identity and habits, you transform healthy behaviors from one-time tasks into enduring routines that reflect who you are. Each of these mindset shifts reinforces the others; together, they create a powerful, positive cycle. You become a person who enjoys the journey of wellness, who sees challenges as part of the process, who doesn't burn out because you're going at your own wise pace, and who ultimately achieves results that last. This is the anti-hustle health plan in action – a genius kind of "laziness" where you put your effort into the mental game upfront so that everything else becomes easier. Master your mindset, and you master your ability to get fit, stay sane, and actually enjoy your life, for good.

Chapter 10

Putting It All Together – Your Anti-Hustle Health Plan

After exploring mindset shifts, gentle movement, nourishing nutrition, restorative rest, and other pillars of wellness throughout this book, you've gathered a toolkit of practices. Now it's time to assemble those pieces into a flexible plan that suits you. Think of it as building your own wellness blueprint – one that honors your unique life rather than forcing you into a one-size-fits-all regimen. In this chapter, we'll craft a personalized "anti-hustle" health plan that you actually enjoy. It will incorporate tiny but powerful steps, emphasize sustainable habits, and remain adaptable as life ebbs and flows. The goal is to help you get fit and stay sane without burning out, so you can truly enjoy your life's moments along the way.

Design Your Personal Plan

Designing your personal plan starts with accepting that there is no universal formula for wellness. Research confirms that a generic one-size-fits-all approach is insufficient for sustaining healthy habits. What works wonders for someone else might not mesh with your schedule, body, or preferences – and that's okay. Instead of following a pre-packaged program to the letter, you'll mix-and-match practices from earlier chapters that resonated with you the most. The anti-hustle approach is all about personalization and listening to your own needs.

Begin by reflecting on what *clicked* for you in each area we covered. Maybe in the movement chapter you discovered you love walking in nature more than high-intensity workouts. In nutrition, perhaps you found a simple breakfast tweak that made you feel energized. From the mindset or rest chapters, you might recall a boundary-setting strategy or a nighttime ritual that helped you relax. List these favorite ideas and habits – they are the building blocks of your custom plan.

Next, fit those pieces into your life's puzzle. Look at your daily and weekly routine and identify where these habits can naturally slot in. If mornings are hectic, an evening stretch or a cup of herbal tea before bed might work better for you than a 5am workout. If you have a flexible lunch break, that could be a perfect time for a brisk walk or a brief breathing exercise. The beauty of a personal plan is that it molds around *your* life, rather than making you bend your life around a rigid program.

Keep it simple and enjoyable. It's tempting to try to "do it all," but remember – we're ditching the hustle mentality. Quality beats quantity. A few meaningful practices you can stick with will beat an overwhelming checklist that leaves you burnt out. Trust that small, consistent actions chosen by you will add up over time. When you enjoy the process, you're far more likely to keep going. In fact, that positive feeling is not a superficial bonus – it's a core feature of this plan. Enjoyment fuels consistency, and consistency fuels results.

Go ahead and write down your personal health plan. It could be in a journal, a note on your phone, or a chart on your wall – whatever makes it feel real for you. Describe the handful of habits you've chosen in clear, friendly language. Think of this as a living document that can evolve, not a strict contract. For now, celebrate that you are *intentionally* crafting a wellness lifestyle tailored to yourself. This is a major departure from cookie-cutter programs. It's empowering because it makes you the expert on your own life.

By designing a personal plan, you're essentially saying: "I choose what works for me, and I let go of what doesn't." That mindset is liberating. Your health journey is no longer about grinding through someone else's routine or feeling guilty for not following the "perfect" plan. Instead, you're free to embrace habits that fit your personality and circumstances. This individualized approach sets you up for success because it builds on your strengths and interests. When a plan aligns with who you are, it becomes sustainable – even *fun*.

Also, remember that nothing in your plan is mandatory just because some expert or trend says so. If you hate running, then running doesn't belong in your plan – perhaps dancing, biking, or gardening gets you moving in ways you enjoy. If you despise kale, you don't have to eat it – maybe bell peppers or berries make you happy. The point of personalization is to choose healthy habits that suit *you*, not to shoehorn yourself into someone else's routine. There's no one "right" way – the right way is the one that you'll actually do and feel good doing.

Tiny Steps, Big Changes

Now that you have the outline of your anti-hustle health plan, how do you start implementing it? The answer is: take tiny steps. Grand, overnight makeovers might sound exciting, but in reality they often lead to overwhelm. The "lazy genius" way recognizes that small, achievable steps can snowball into big changes over time. In fact, consistently making modest improvements can yield remarkable results due to the power of compounding. (In fact, if you improve by 1% each day for a year, you end up roughly 37 times better by the end!) Improving by just 1% every day can make you dramatically better over months, whereas attempting a 100% change in one go is usually unsustainable.

For example, Britain's cycling team famously applied the philosophy of "marginal gains," improving every tiny thing by 1%. These small tweaks – better seat comfort, cleaner bike tires, improved sleep for athletes – added up to Olympic gold medals. The lesson? Tiny steps matter. You don't need an Olympic goal to use this approach in your life. It means focusing on one small habit at a time, trusting that mini-wins will compound into major improvements in your fitness and well-being.

Let's lay out a sample "lazy genius" 4-week kickstart to show how gradual additions can lead to significant change. This is just an example – you can adjust it to fit your chosen habits:

- **Week 1:** Add a 10-minute walk to your lunch break each day. It could be around your building or a quick stroll outside. Even a brief daily walk can lift your mood and get your blood flowing. In fact, researchers estimate that adding just 10 minutes of brisk walking per day is associated with about a 7% reduction in yearly mortality risk – a longevity boost from a tiny habit.

- **Week 2:** Go to bed 30 minutes earlier than usual. Use that extra half-hour for additional sleep or a calming wind-down routine. Many of us are chronically underslept, and a little more pillow time can make a big difference. One study with college students found that about 40 extra minutes of sleep per night led to less daytime sleepiness and even lowered their blood pressure. In other words, a modest bump in sleep can yield measurable health improvements.

- **Week 3:** Introduce one nutrition upgrade. For example, add an extra serving of vegetables to one meal, or swap a sugary afternoon snack for a piece of fruit or nuts. Pick a *single* food change that feels very doable. Small changes in diet, maintained over time, can improve your health more than any drastic crash diet. The key is choosing something you don't mind (maybe even enjoy) – like discovering a new favorite smoothie or seasoning veggies in a tasty way. These tiny tweaks to your eating habits, repeated daily, will add up.

- **Week 4:** Add a 5-minute mindful break each day. This could be gentle stretching, deep breathing, journaling one grateful thought, or simply stepping outside for fresh air. By week 4, you've incorporated movement, sleep, and nutrition habits; now include a quick stress-relief or mindset practice. Even a few minutes of mindfulness or relaxation can reduce stress and improve your focus for the rest of the day.

By the end of these four weeks, you've layered four small habits into your routine: walking, getting more sleep, a nutrition tweak, and a daily mindful pause. None of these required extreme effort or drastic schedule changes – yet together they create a positive ripple effect. You might notice you have more energy, better sleep quality, improved mood, or even that your clothes fit a bit looser. Equally important, you've built confidence by proving to yourself that progress is possible even with a busy schedule. By focusing on one change at a time, you avoided overwhelm and burnout. As one habits expert put it, we tend to overestimate the impact of big sudden actions and underestimate the power of small daily improvements. Those tiny steps truly lead to big changes when you give them time to accumulate.

Accountability and Adaptability

Sticking with your personal plan is the next challenge – and we want to do it without sliding back into hustle-mode stress. Two key principles will help you stay on track gently: accountability and adaptability.

First, accountability. Humans are social creatures; we often do better when we feel supported and when someone is cheering us on. But the *type* of accountability matters. We're not looking for a drill sergeant or guilt trips. Aim for gentle accountability that encourages you. One great option is to find a wellness buddy. This could be a friend or colleague who also wants a balanced approach to health. Agree to check in with each other regularly – not to police mistakes, but to share wins and challenges. For example, you might text each other a couple of times a week about your progress ("Took my walk today and feel great" or "Tough day, only managed a short walk"). Knowing someone cares can motivate you when inertia hits. You might even make it a friendly challenge – for example, see if you and your buddy can each hit a certain number of steps in a week and then celebrate together when you do. Social support has been shown to strengthen commitment to exercise and healthy habits. In fact, not having a workout partner is a common barrier to exercise that many people report. A buddy helps fill that gap by providing camaraderie and accountability in a positive way.

If a real-life buddy isn't available, use a journal or a habit-tracking app as your accountability partner. Checking off a habit each day or jotting a brief note about what you did can give you a satisfying sense of accomplishment. Self-monitoring is a proven behavior-change aid – one study found that people who kept daily food records lost twice as much weight as those who kept no records, simply because writing things down made them mindful of their actions. In your case, you might keep a simple log of your new habits: mark on a calendar each day you do your walk or get to bed on time, or write one sentence about how you felt after completing a habit. The act of tracking reinforces the behavior and gives you a reason to celebrate small wins. Just remember to keep it friendly and use the log to encourage yourself, not to beat yourself up on off-days.

While using accountability, guard against turning it into pressure. If an app's reminders stress you out, dial them back. If you skip a journal entry, don't worry. The goal is to support yourself, not create a new source of guilt. This is the anti-hustle plan – shame and harshness have no place here.

Equally important is adaptability. Life will throw curveballs, and even the best plan needs adjusting sometimes. The old all-or-nothing approach would have us think a lapse means total failure – but not in this plan. Here, if things change, you change the plan (not abandon it). Remind yourself that your plan is a flexible, *living* document – you can tweak it whenever needed. Think of it as a roadmap rather than a rigid decree.

How does adaptability work? Suppose you've been doing your 10-minute lunch walks faithfully, but this week a big work deadline eats up your lunch break. In a rigid mindset, you might feel like you "failed" and then give up exercising that week. With adaptability, you adjust: maybe you do a 5-minute stretch at your desk, or take a short walk in the morning instead. If you're traveling or dealing with a family crisis, you might temporarily scale down to just one or two core habits (say, prioritizing sleep and staying hydrated) until you can resume the others. Adjust the plan instead of throwing it out.

One useful mantra is "never miss twice". It's okay to miss a habit one day – life happens! – but try to get back on track the next day so that a one-day slip doesn't turn into a new pattern. For example, if you skipped your walk today, shrug it off and make a point to walk tomorrow. By catching yourself after one miss, you prevent a small lapse from snowballing into a slump.

Above all, practice self-compassion when things don't go perfectly. Talk to yourself the way you'd talk to a friend who hit a snag. Instead of, "I'm so lazy, I blew it," try, "I've been doing well, one off day doesn't erase my progress. I can restart tomorrow." This kind of kind self-talk isn't just feel-good fluff – research shows that responding to setbacks with self-compassion helps people persevere with their goals rather than quit. By forgiving yourself for being human, you empower yourself to bounce back faster. So if work heats up or you get derailed, be flexible and gentle. Maintain the basics you can, and when the storm passes, ramp back up. Adaptability ensures that wellness stays sustainable through life's ups and downs, without the drama of "falling off the wagon."

Enjoying the Journey

As you put it all together – your personal plan, tiny steps, accountability, and adaptability – keep sight of the big picture: a health journey that enhances your life, not one that *is* your life. The core of this plan is enjoyment. Why? Because a wellness plan you enjoy is one you'll actually stick with, and ultimately the whole point is to be happier and healthier, not just hit some number on a scale.

Think back to Chapter 1. We met the burnout mindset – the overachiever running on fumes, trying to do everything "right" and feeling miserable. Now you've flipped that script. Armed with science-backed insights and a kinder approach, you're improving your fitness in a way that fuels you rather than drains you. You're pursuing health in a manner that makes you happier, not stressed out. That's a huge transformation from the start of this journey.

Enjoyment isn't a luxury here – it's a strategy. Traditional hustle culture might preach "no pain, no gain," but you've seen that joy is actually a powerful fuel for gain – when you like what you're doing, you naturally keep doing it. When you genuinely enjoy your activities, you need far less willpower to do them. Studies even confirm that enjoyment is a strong predictor of sticking with exercise routines. By now, you've chosen forms of movement and self-care that you *like* – maybe it's morning yoga with music, or walking the dog at sunset, or cooking a fun new recipe. Because these habits bring you satisfaction (or at least a sense of peace and accomplishment), they're not chores on your to-do list; they're welcome parts of your day. That changes everything. Instead of dreading a workout, you might find you're looking forward to that break in your day. Instead of feeling guilty about food, you're enjoying meals that both taste good and nourish you. This positive emotional feedback is powerful fuel.

Ironically, by not obsessing over outcomes and by focusing on the process, those health outcomes tend to improve naturally. You might suddenly realize your energy is higher, you're less anxious, or your jeans fit more loosely. Perhaps your doctor will smile at your next check-up because your numbers moved in the right direction. These are fantastic wins – and you achieved them without punishing yourself or living at the gym. You've proven that you can get results while living a balanced, enjoyable life.

Ultimately, the anti-hustle health plan is about living better day by day. It's about *quality of life*. Yes, you're getting fitter, but more importantly, you're savoring life's moments more fully. You have the energy to play with your kids or pursue hobbies because you're not burned out from extreme regimens. You can be present with loved ones because you're not constantly stressed about your wellness checklist. By embracing this philosophy, you've made wellness a part of your life rather than a ruthless project. Your life is actually *bigger* now – you have more energy and freedom – instead of wellness making your life feel smaller or restricted.

As you move forward, keep listening to your body and mind. Your plan will continue to evolve – that's a good thing. Stay open to trying new small habits and retiring ones that no longer serve you. There is no finish line; this is a lifelong dance with your well-being. But with the skills and mindset you have now, you can trust yourself to navigate it.

In the end, remember to celebrate how far you've come. You chose a kinder path in a world that often pushes us to grind harder. You learned that getting fit, staying sane, and actually enjoying life can all go together – and you made it happen. That is the ultimate win. Even if you once felt like an exhausted overachiever or someone who hated the very idea of working out, you've now proven there's a gentler way to wellness that truly works for you. So here's to your anti-hustle health journey ahead: may it be sustainable, rewarding, and filled with joy every step of the way.

Epilogue

As you close this book, remember, wellness doesn't have to be a race. It's not about relentless hustle, impossible standards, or grueling hours at the gym. It's about finding the rhythm that suits you, the path that doesn't demand your soul in exchange for health. You've learned that small actions, done consistently, can transform your life. A few minutes of movement here, a mindful meal there, and the occasional restful pause can create a life that feels both full and sustainable.

The journey to health isn't linear, and it certainly isn't a one-size-fits-all formula. Your wellness plan is yours to define, based on what feels right for your body, mind, and lifestyle. There will be days when you feel unstoppable and others when you need to slow down. Both are okay. Embrace the messy, imperfect process and celebrate the wins—no matter how small. The key is progress, not perfection.

So, take a deep breath, step back, and reflect on how far you've come. Each change, no matter how tiny, adds up over time. You've created the space for joy, for balance, and for a life that's both healthy and enjoyable. Wellness is a marathon, not a sprint. And you've learned to run it on your terms, at your pace.

You're not bound by society's definition of success or the endless pressure to do more. You are free to live your life—on your own terms, at your own pace. Keep moving forward, keep laughing, and above all, keep enjoying the ride. You've earned it.